T0362522

ORTHOPEDIC CLINICS OF NORTH AMERICA

www.orthopedic.theclinics.com

Intraoperative Challenges

January 2024 • Volume 55 • Number 1

Editor-in-Chief
FREDERICK M. AZAR

Editorial Board
MICHAEL J. BEEBE
CLAYTON C. BETTIN
TYLER J. BROLIN
JAMES H. CALANDRUCCIO
CHRISTOPHER T. COSGROVE
MARCUS C. FORD
BENJAMIN J. GREAR
BENJAMIN M. MAUCK[†]
WILLIAM M. MIHALKO
BENJAMIN SHEFFER
KIRK M. THOMPSON
WILLIAM J. WELLER

ELSEVIER

1600 John F. Kennedy Boulevard • Suite 1800 • Philadelphia, Pennsylvania, 19103-2899.

http://www.orthopedic.theclinics.com

ORTHOPEDIC CLINICS OF NORTH AMERICA Volume 55, Number 1
January 2024 ISSN 0030-5898, ISBN-13: 978-0-443-18421-5

Editor: Megan Ashdown
Developmental Editor: Shivank Joshi

Orthopedic Clinics of North America (ISSN 0030-5898) is published quarterly by Elsevier Inc., 360 Park Avenue South, New York, NY 10010-1710. Months of issue are January, April, July, and October. Business and Editorial Offices: 1600 John F. Kennedy Blvd., Suite 1800, Philadelphia, PA 19103-2899. Customer Service Office: 3251 Riverport Lane, Maryland Heights, MO 63043. Periodicals postage paid at New York, NY and additional mailing offices. Subscription prices are $368.00 per year for (US individuals), $433.00 per year (Canadian individuals), $511.00 per year (international individuals), $100.00 per year (US students), $100.00 per year for (Canadian students), $220.00 per year for (international students). For institutional access pricing please contact Customer Service via the contact information below. Foreign air speed delivery is included in all *Clinics* subscription prices. All prices are subject to change without notice. **POSTMASTER:** Send change of address to *Orthopedic Clinics of North America*, **Elsevier Health Sciences Division, Subscription Customer Service, 3251 Riverport Lane, Maryland Heights, MO 63043. Customer Service (orders, claims, online, change of address): Elsevier Health Sciences Division, Subscription Customer Service, 3251 Riverport Lane, Maryland Heights, MO 63043. Tel: 1-800-654-2452 (U.S. and Canada); 314-447-8871 (outside U.S. and Canada). Fax: 314-447-8029. E-mail:** journalscustomerservice-usa@elsevier.com **(for print support);** journalsonlinesupport-usa@elsevier.com **(for online support).**

Reprints. For copies of 100 or more, of articles in this publication, please contact the Commercial Reprints Department, Elsevier Inc., 360 Park Avenue South, New York, NY 10010-1710. Tel.: 212-633-3874; Fax: 212-633-3820; E-mail: reprints@elsevier.com.

Orthopedic Clinics of North America is covered in *MEDLINE/PubMed* (*Index Medicus*), *Cinahl, Excerpta Medica,* and *Cumulative Index to Nursing and Allied Health Literature.*

EDITORIAL BOARD

CONTRIBUTORS

EDITOR

FREDERICK M. AZAR, MD
Professor, Department of Orthopaedic
Surgery & Biomedical Engineering, University
of Tennessee-Campbell Clinic; Chief-of-Staff,
Campbell Clinic, Inc, Memphis, Tennessee,
USA

AUTHORS

ZACHARY ABERMAN, MD
Fellow Orthopedic Surgery, Adult
Reconstruction, Lenox Hill Hospital, New York
City, NY, USA

C. LOWRY BARNES, MD
Department of Orthopaedics, University of
Arkansas for Medical Sciences, Little Rock,
Arkansas, USA

JARED A. BELL, MD
Hand and Upper Extremity Fellowship,
University of Tennessee-Campbell Clinic,
Memphis, Tennessee, USA

AMIT K. BHANDUTIA, MD
Assistant Professor, Louisiana State University
Health Sciences Center Orthopaedic and
Spine Surgery, New Orleans, Louisiana,
USA

MICHAEL BOLOGNESI, MD
Orthopedist, Division of Orthopedic Surgery,
Duke University, Durham, North Carolina, USA

NICHOLAS M. BROWN, MD
Associate Professor, Loyola University Medical
Center, Maywood, Illinois, USA

JAMES H. CALANDRUCCIO, MD
Associate Professor, Campbell Clinic
Department of Orthopedic Surgery, University
of Tennessee Health Science Center,
Germantown, Tennessee, USA

TYLER E. CALKINS, MD
Orthopedic Surgeon, Departments of
Orthopaedic Surgery and Biomedical

Engineering, University of Tennessee-
Campbell Clinic, Memphis, Tennessee, USA

DANIELLE CHUN, MD
Fellow, Adult Reconstruction, Medical School
Northwestern University, Division of
Orthopedic Surgery, Durham, North Carolina,
USA

SETH R. COPE, MD
Departments of Orthopaedic Surgery and
Biomedical Engineering, University of
Tennessee-Campbell Clinic, Memphis,
Tennessee, USA

KEVIN J. CRONIN, MD
Florida Orthopaedic Institute, Tampa, Florida,
USA; Assistant Professor, Department of
Orthopaedic Surgery and Sports Medicine,
University of South Florida, Florida
Orthopaedic Institute, Temple Terrace,
Florida, USA

MATTHEW DARLOW, MD
Orthopedic Surgeon, Louisiana State
University Health Sciences Center
Orthopaedic Surgery Resident, New Orleans,
Louisiana, USA

MALCOLM DEBAUN, MD
Assistant Professor, Division of Orthopedic
Surgery, Duke University, Durham, North
Carolina, USA

KATHERINE DONG, MD
Orthopedic Surgery Resident, Louisiana State
University Health Sciences Center
Orthopaedic Surgery Resident, New Orleans,
Louisiana, USA

ANDREAS FONTALIS, MD, MSc (Res),
MRCS (Eng)
Trauma and Orthopaedic Surgery Specialist
Registrar at The Percivall Pott Orthopaedic
Rotation, London, United Kingdom

LIZ FORD, DO
Orthopedic Surgery Resident, Inspira Health
Network, Vineland, New Jersey, USA

MARCUS C. FORD, MD
Assistant Professor, University of Tennessee
HSC-Campbell Clinic, Memphis, Tennessee,
USA

MARK A. FRANKLE, MD
Professor, Department of Orthopaedic
Surgery and Sports Medicine, University of
South Florida, Florida Orthopaedic Institute,
Temple Terrace, Florida, USA

JOSHUA L. GARY, MD
Chief of Orthopedic Trauma Service,
Associate Professor of Clinical Orthopedic
Surgery, Clinical Scholar, Department of
Orthopedic Surgery, Keck School of Medicine
of USC, Los Angeles, California, USA

DANIEL GELVEZ, MD
Resident PGY2, Louisiana State University
Health Sciences Center Orthopaedic Surgery
Resident, New Orleans, Louisiana, USA

JAMES GERMANO, MD
Chair of Orthopedics, Long Island Valley
Stream Hospital Northwell Health, Valley
Stream, New York, USA

DIA ELDEAN GIEBALY, MBChB, MSc,
FRCS (Tr&Orth), MBA
Department of Trauma and Orthopaedic
Surgery, University College Hospital, Division
of Surgery and Interventional Science,
University College London, London, United
Kingdom

CHRISTOPHER E. GROSS, MD
Professor, Department of Orthopaedic
Surgery, Medical University of South Carolina,
Charleston, South Carolina, USA

AKRAM A. HABIBI, MD
Department of Orthopedic Surgery, NYU
Langone Health, New York, New York, USA

FARES S. HADDAD, BSc, MD(Res),
MCh(Orth), FRCS(Orth), FFSEM
Department of Trauma and Orthopaedic
Surgery, University College Hospital, Division
of Surgery and Interventional Science,
University College London, London, United
Kingdom

SHANIL HANSJEE, BA, BM, BCh
Fellow, Department of Trauma and
Orthopaedic Surgery, University College
Hospital, London, United Kingdom

IAN G. HASEGAWA, MD
Orthopedic Trauma Fellow, Department of
Orthopedic Surgery, Keck School of Medicine
of USC, Los Angeles, California,
USA

MICHAEL D. HELLMAN, MD
Orthopedic Surgery Specialist, Rockhill
Orthopaedic Specialists, Lees Summit,
Missouri, USA

SYDNEY M. HODGESON, MD
Orthopedic Surgery Resident, Department of
Orthopaedics, University of Arkansas for
Medical Sciences, Little Rock, Arkansas, USA

NICHOLAS F. JAMES, MD
Assistant Professor, Department of
Orthopedic Surgery, University of Florida
Health Jacksonville, Jacksonville, Florida,
USA

STERLING KRAMER, DO
Fellow, Campbell Clinic, Campbell
Foundation, Memphis, Tennessee, USA

NITHYA LINGAMPALLI, MD
Resident Physician, Loyola University Medical
Center, Maywood, Illinois, USA

FABIO MANCINO, MD
Department of Trauma and Orthopaedic
Surgery, University College Hospital, London,
United Kingdom

BENJAMIN M. MAUCK, MD
Hand and Upper Extremity Surgery, Campbell
Clinic; Clinical Instructor, Department of
Orthopedic Surgery, University of Tennessee
Health Science Center, Memphis, Tennessee

SIMON C. MEARS, MD, PhD
Professor, Department of Orthopaedics,
College of Medicine at University of Arkansas
for Medical Sciences, Little Rock, Arkansas,
USA

ZACHARY A. MOSHER, MD
Departments of Orthopaedic Surgery and
Biomedical Engineering, University of
Tennessee-Campbell Clinic, Memphis,
Tennessee, USA

CHRISTIAN PEAN, MD, MS
Division of Orthopedic Surgery, Duke
University, Durham, North Carolina, USA

ZACHARY K. PHARR, MD
Departments of Orthopaedic Surgery and
Biomedical Engineering, University of
Tennessee-Campbell Clinic, Memphis,
Tennessee, USA

RICCI PLASTOW, MBChB, FRCS (Eng)
Department of Trauma and Orthopaedic
Surgery, University College Hospital, London,
United Kingdom

KEVIN F. PURCELL, MD, MPH, MS
Division of Orthopedic Surgery, Duke
University, Durham, North Carolina, USA

NATHAN REDLICH, MD
Louisiana State University Health Sciences
Center Orthopaedic Surgery Resident, New
Orleans, Louisiana, USA

SEAN RYAN, MD
Division of Orthopedic Surgery, Duke
University, Durham, North Carolina, USA

RAN SCHWARZKOPF, MD, MSc
Department of Orthopedic Surgery, NYU
Langone Health, New York, New York, USA

DANIEL J. SCOTT, MD, MBA
Associate Professor, Department of
Orthopaedic Surgery, Medical University of
South Carolina, Charleston, South Carolina,
USA

GILES R. SCUDERI, MD
Vice President Orthopedic Service Line,
Northwell Health, Garden City, New York,
USA

THORSTEN SEYLER, MD, PhD
Assistant Professor, Division of Orthopedic
Surgery, Duke University, Durham, North
Carolina, USA

BERJE SHAMMASSIAN, MD
Assistant Professor, Louisiana State University
Health Sciences Center Neurosurgery, New
Orleans, Louisiana, USA

AUSTIN LUKE SHIVER, MD
Pediatric Orthopedic Specialist, Medical
College of Georgia at Augusta University,
Augusta, Georgia, USA

AUSTIN F. SMITH, MD
Orthopaedic Surgeon at Orthopaedic Medical
Group, Florida Orthopaedic Institute, Tampa,
Florida, USA

MARK C. SNODDY, MD
Orthopedist, Medical College of Georgia at
Augusta University, Augusta, Georgia, USA

TATSUYA SOENO, MD
Department of Orthopaedics, University of
Arkansas for Medical Sciences, Little Rock,
Arkansas, USA

JEFFREY B. STAMBOUGH, MD
Department of Orthopaedics, University of
Arkansas for Medical Sciences, Little Rock,
Arkansas, USA

TAYLOR P. STAUFFER, BS
School of Medicine, Duke University, Duke
University Hospital, Durham, North Carolina,
USA

BENJAMIN M. STRONACH, MS, MD
Department of Orthopaedics, University of
Arkansas for Medical Sciences, Little Rock,
Arkansas, USA

DOYLE R. WALLACE, MD
Orthopedic Surgery Specialist, Medical
College of Georgia at Augusta University,
Augusta, Georgia, USA

JED WALSH, DO
Department of Orthopaedic Surgery, Inspira
Health Network, Vineland, New Jersey, USA

WILLIAM J. WELLER, MD
Assistant Professor, Campbell Clinic
Department of Orthopedic Surgery, University
of Tennessee Health Science Center,
Germantown, Tennessee, USA

JONATHON WHITEHEAD, MD
Orthopedic Surgeon, Medical College of
Georgia, Augusta University, Augusta,
Georgia, USA

JESTIN WILLIAMS, MD
Louisiana State University Health Sciences
Center Orthopaedic Surgery Resident, New
Orleans, Louisiana, USA

MATTHEW WOOD, MD
Orthopedist, Medical College of Georgia,
Augusta University, Augusta, Georgia, USA

CONTENTS

Total knee arthroplasty (TKA) is a widely accepted surgical procedure for managing end-stage knee osteoarthritis. Among the various TKA techniques, kinematic alignment has gained increasing popularity as it can potentially restore a more natural joint function. However, despite its theoretical advantages, kinematic total knee replacement presents several operative challenges that necessitate a thorough understanding and analysis of patient-specific anatomy during surgical planning and execution. This review article aims to critically evaluate the operative challenges associated with kinematic TKA and explore potential strategies to optimize surgical outcomes. The challenges encompass multiple aspects including patient selection, preoperative planning, bone cuts, soft tissue balancing, and component positioning.

▶ Video content accompanies this article at http://www.orthopedic.theclinics.com.

The introduction of new surgical technology highlights appreciable concerns; robotic arthroplasty is no exception. Acquiring comprehensive understanding of the robotic technology to avoid complications during surgery and devising troubleshooting strategies to overcome potential difficulties is of paramount importance. Troubleshooting algorithms depend on the stage of the procedure and problem encountered, such as loosening of the pins or array, registration or verification problems, or malfunctioning of the device, which is rare. This article aims to outline reproducible workflows and solutions for troubleshooting during robotic-arm assisted total hip arthroplasty and total knee arthroplasty.

Medial pivot total knee arthroplasty implants are designed to function in a similar manner to that of the native knee with a relatively fixed medial center of rotation and a less conforming lateral compartment that follows an arcuate path. Medial pivot implants in total knee arthroplasty have increased in popularity with many companies offering medial pivot or retrofitted medial congruent implants, and there are variations between the various medial pivot and medial congruent implants. Existing literature on medial pivot implants have demonstrated high survivorship and patient outcomes. More studies are needed to compare newer medial pivot implants with each other and with retrofitted medial congruent implants.

A review article summarizes the existing literature on intraoperative injury to medial collateral ligament (MCL) during total knee arthroplasty (TKA), methods of fixation, repair, and the outcomes after these injuries. The options for increasing implant constraint and repair of the MCL injury are discussed with the potential indications for each. There is also a review of risk factors for MCL injury during TKA to help anticipate potential issues preoperatively. The proper use of retractors during total knee replacement is also discussed with a focus on careful protection of the MCL during surgery.

Trauma

Achieving high-quality intraoperative imaging is crucial for successful pelvic ring and acetabular fracture surgery, yet it remains clinically challenging. Due to the complex anatomy of the pelvic ring and acetabulum, it is necessary to obtain multiple images oriented in different planes to reliably confirm reduction accuracy and implant positioning. Intraoperative image quality can be compromised by factors such as patient body habitus, bowel gas, abdominal packing, contrast dye, and nonstandardized language between surgeon and radiology technician. This article reviews common intraoperative imaging challenges encountered during pelvic ring and acetabular fracture surgery, while providing practical and evidence-based solutions and prevention strategies.

Pediatrics

Spinal cord injury is one of the most feared complications in spinal deformity surgery. The surgeon must be vigilant of direct and indirect sources of injury at all points during surgery. The incidence of complications has greatly decreased with the ability to monitor the motor and sensory pathways. Changes in signaling of these pathways provide context for what the insult is, and how to correct it before it becomes irreversible. There are well-established protocols that provide an algorithmic response to changes that can help all in the room determine the source of injury, and the appropriate reaction.

Shoulder and Elbow

As the incidence of shoulder arthroplasty continues to rise, encountering significant glenoid bone loss in the primary and revision setting is becoming a common occurrence. To effectively treat these difficult scenarios, surgeons must understand the common patterns of glenoid bone loss and be aware of the various techniques available for treatment. Understanding bone loss requires careful pre-operative evaluation with appropriate imaging and pre-operative planning software. Treatment algorithms consist of primary anatomic and reverse arthroplasty as well as the use of allograft or autograft bone grafting, augmented glenoid components, specialized surgical techniques, or custom implant designs. Ultimately, good outcomes are able to be obtained with various techniques when applied to the appropriate clinical situation.

Hand and Wrist

Distal radius fractures are some of the most common injuries encountered in orthopedics and require careful consideration when determining the appropriate treatment options. These fractures can be difficult injuries to treat surgically based on a large variability of fracture patterns, bone quality, and anatomy. It is important to understand the potential pitfalls associated with the treatment of difficult distal radius fractures to prevent avoidable complications. Some of these pitfalls include but are not limited to appropriate surgical exposure and soft tissue handling, provisional reduction, fixation type, and augmentation of fracture fixation.

A wide array of intraoperative issues can arise during surgery involving the hand and upper extremity. An understanding of the common pitfalls within hand surgery may help practicing hand surgeons circumvent such issues. Within this manuscript, we first identify problems with the increasingly popular technique of wide-awake local anesthesia no tourniquet (WALANT). Achieving appropriate hemostasis and anesthetic can be bothersome, especially for procedures proximal to the distal palmar crease. We discuss our local anesthetic timing and concentrations to help mitigate such issues, as well as other problems that may arise in WALANT procedures. There also lies a barrier in connecting the traumatized patient to care in the outpatient/ambulatory setting. Additionally, the polytraumatized patient increases the complexity of care coordination for not just the hand surgeon, but all surgical providers involved. The order in which multidisciplinary surgical procedures are performed is influenced by both the complexity of the patient's case as well as the institution's current protocol. All academic institutions are faced with challenges in providing optimal intraoperative education to trainees. We acknowledge that there should be a balance between the attending surgeon executing key portions of the procedure and the trainee gaining the appropriate hands-on experience. This manuscript elaborates on the issues of intraoperative education provided to residents and anecdotal methods that may help overcome such challenges. Resources within hand surgery can often be limited and become particularly problematic in the operative setting. Specific examples include but are not limited to the lack of dedicated teams, inability to obtain appropriate intraoperative imaging, access to appropriate hardware, and intraoperative complications in an ambulatory surgery center setting.

Foot and Ankle

Intraoperative complications during total ankle replacement (TAR) can be devastating. As surgeons' experience with total ankles grow and surgical techniques are refined, intraoperative complications, such as fractures, can still occur. Surgeons must be able to recognize a problem, identify the options to remediate, and then execute a solution readily. Unfortunately, given the heterogeneity of TAR outcome studies, it is difficult to garner the true incidence of complications in the peri-operative period following ankle replacements. The purpose of this review is to focus on perioperative fractures during TAR. Fractures can occur intraoperatively and postoperatively as stress fractures or post-operative trauma.

Spine

Vertebral artery injury (VAI) is a serious and potentially life-threatening injury that is encountered with trauma to the cervical spine and less frequently during surgery. VAI can occur during either anterior or posterior cervical approaches or instrumentation and often involves anomalous courses of the artery. Although the incidence is rare, serious consequences including fistula formation, thrombosis, pseudoaneurysm development, cerebral ischemia, hemorrhage, and death may occur. Management of VAI can be divided into prevention, including review of preoperative imaging with knowledge of the anatomic course, utilization of surgical landmarks intraoperatively, and prompt recognition and management when injury is encountered.

INTRAOPERATIVE CHALLENGES

PREFACE

Intraoperative Challenges

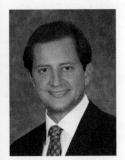

Frederick M. Azar, MD
Editor

Orthopedic surgeons face challenges on a daily basis, but none more so than during surgery. Although basic surgical techniques are standard to some extent, each patient is an individual, with a unique anatomy, body habitus, condition, and comorbidities, and requires individualized treatment; every technique requires fine-tuning to meet distinct needs. Surgery without the risk of complication does not exist regardless of the best laid plans. There are general risks of surgery and technique-specific risks, and some surgeries have a high probability of adverse events so much so that protocols have been put in place to avoid or treat problems as they arise. This issue of *Orthopedic Clinics of North America* explores some of the intraoperative challenges and complications encountered in total joint arthroplasty, upper- and lower-extremity fracture surgery, and spine surgery. The general consensus of these articles appears to be that careful patient selection; appropriate preoperative evaluation, including a review of risk factors and imaging; proper implant choice; a clear understanding of anatomy, injury

morphology, and the surgical procedure as well as its pitfalls; and meticulous surgical technique are necessary to lessen the chance of an avoidable complication. Much research has been done on avoiding iatrogenic injury, and surgeons must make every effort to circumvent such events. Nonetheless, when a complication does occur during surgery, and it will despite exquisite care exercised by the surgical team, it is helpful to have a mitigation strategy in place to optimize the final outcome. Management options for common complications, such as intraoperative fracture during joint reconstructive procedures, are provided, and fixation strategies are offered. Although reducing the risk of complications is a top priority, complications are not the only orthopedic challenges with which orthopedic surgeons must contend. Some injuries are inherently difficult to treat. One such example is total shoulder revision in the face of glenoid bone loss. Regardless of treatment, decreased clinical outcomes may result in this scenario. Procedures such as kinematic total knee replacement (TKA), medial pivot TKA, and robotic TKA all have

Orthop Clin N Am 55 (2024) xv–xvi
https://doi.org/10.1016/j.ocl.2023.09.003
0030-5898/24/© 2023 Published by Elsevier Inc.

their unique issues as well. In trauma there is the challenge of intraoperative imaging in pelvic ring and acetabular fracture surgery. The challenge lies in the limited ability of two-dimensional fluoroscopy to reliably confirm reduction accuracy. Some fracture patterns, such as occurs in the distal radius, also require careful consideration, with treatment depending on bone quality and injury characteristics. It is incumbent upon the surgeon to provide the patient with the best chance for a good outcome by preparing thoroughly for the procedure. We would like to thank the authors in this issue, who have provided excellent reviews and offered practical solutions and best practices for challenging procedures and complications.

Dr Azar discloses the following outside of this work: Pfizer; Zimmer; Elsevier; JSES; Orthopedic Clinics; Wolters Kluwer; St. Jude; ABOS; AJSM.

Frederick M. Azar, MD
Campbell Clinic, Inc
University of Tennessee-Campbell Clinic
Department of Orthopaedic Surgery & Biomedical
Engineering
1211 Union Avenue
Suite 510
Memphis, TN 38104, USA

E-mail address:
fazar@campbellclinic.com

Safety of Outpatient Total Hip Arthroplasty Performed in Patients 65 Years of Age and Older in an Ambulatory Surgery Center

Zachary A. Mosher, MD[a,b], Tyler E. Calkins, MD[a,b], Seth R. Cope, MD[a,b], Zachary K. Pharr, MD[a,b], Marcus C. Ford, MD[a,b],*

KEYWORDS

- Same-day discharge • Outpatient total hip arthroplasty • Ambulatory surgery center • Geriatric
- Safety

KEY POINTS

- Studies on the safety profile of same-day discharge total hip arthroplasty (THA) in patients ≥ 65 years of age are lacking.
- A retrospective review of 69 patients (≥65 years) who underwent same-day discharge primary THA in 2 ambulatory surgery centers was performed to determine safety and complications.
- Sixty-six of 69 patients (96%) met same-day discharge goals with a mean facility duration of 8 hours and 45 minutes.
- One intraoperative complication occurred that required transport to a hospital for transfusion and 2 patients required overnight stay at the ambulatory surgery center for the prolonged effect of spinal anesthesia as well as urinary retention.
- Patients ≥ 65 years having outpatient THA in an ambulatory surgery center can safely undergo planned same-day discharge after appropriate preoperative evaluation, patient selection, and patient education.

INTRODUCTION

Total hip arthroplasty (THA) has evolved to include planned same-day and next-day discharge.[1–3] This has led to an increase in outpatient total joint arthroplasty (TJA) with improved patient satisfaction, cost-effectiveness, and equivalent safety compared to inpatient procedures.[4–8] However, the increase in outpatient THA has mostly been limited to younger patients due to reimbursement and safety concerns in elderly in the United States.[9,10] THA was on the "inpatient-only" Medicare insurance list until January 1, 2020, when it was approved as an outpatient surgery in hospitals. On January 1, 2021, it was approved for ambulatory surgery centers.[11–13]

With THA in older patients historically being performed in hospitals, studies evaluating outpatient THA in this patient population are lacking, with few studies investigating its safety in ambulatory surgery centers.[14–16] Only one study specifically evaluated same-day discharge

[a] Department of Orthopaedic Surgery, University of Tennessee-Campbell Clinic, 1211 Union Avenue, Suite 510, Memphis, TN 38014, USA; [b] Department of Biomedical Engineering, University of Tennessee-Campbell Clinic, 1211 Union Avenue, Suite 510, Memphis, TN 38014, USA
* Corresponding author. 1400 South Germantown Road, Germantown, TN 38138
E-mail address: mford@campbellclinic.com

Orthop Clin N Am 55 (2024) 1–7
https://doi.org/10.1016/j.ocl.2023.05.009
0030-5898/24/© 2023 Elsevier Inc. All rights reserved.

after THA in older-aged patients, but it was done in a hospital.[17]

The purpose of this review was to determine if same-day discharge of patients over the age of 65 years undergoing THA at an ambulatory surgery center is a safe practice.

MATERIALS AND METHODS

After institutional review board approval and a waiver of informed consent, all patients who had THA in two ambulatory surgery centers from June, 2013 to June, 2020 were identified via medical records. Patients younger than 65 years of age on the day of surgery and those with less than 90-day follow-up were excluded. Surgical candidacy was based on a modified version of the criteria published by Fournier and colleagues and Toy and colleagues (Fig. 1).[9,10]

Operative Procedure
A direct anterior approach or posterolateral approach to THA was used based on surgeon preference. Hypotensive spinal anesthesia was used unless contraindicated or technically unfeasible. Local capsular and soft-tissue injections were used, including liposomal bupivacaine or a multimodal injection consisting of ropivacaine with epinephrine, ketorolac, and morphine.[18]

Postoperative Protocol
All patients were given oral multimodal pain control and ambulated with a rolling walker under the supervision of a physical therapist or trained registered nurse. If patients were unable to void within 2 hours postoperatively, they were given bethanechol orally. If this continued beyond 8 hours, an indwelling catheter was placed and outpatient urology follow-up scheduled within 3 to 5 days. Discharge criteria were ability to eat without nausea/vomiting, pain control with oral medications, mobilization without orthostatic hypotension or syncope, stable vital signs at rest and after activity, and voiding control. Patients were discharged home and scheduled for physical therapy within 3 days after surgery.

Outcome Variables
Demographic information, preoperative comorbidities (cardiac disease, pulmonary disease, anemia, hypertension, diabetes mellitus, obstructive sleep apnea, venous thromboembolism, cancer, hepatitis, renal disease, and mood disorders), tobacco and alcohol use, day-of-surgery and intraoperative information, and 90-day postoperative outcomes, were collected. A cumulative calculation of preoperative comorbidities, tobacco use, and alcohol abuse was obtained, with the presence of each comorbidity or social factor being worth 1 point. American Society of Anesthesiologists (ASA) Physical Status Classification was delineated by the anesthesia provider preoperatively.

Surgery-specific data (operative approach, surgeon, facility, and primary diagnosis) were recorded. Intraoperative and day-of surgery data, including anesthesia, estimated blood loss, operative time, postoperative ambulation distance, time to ambulation, postoperative facility duration (time from procedure completion to discharge), and total facility duration (time of arrival into the preoperative area to time of discharge), were recorded. Visual analog scale (VAS) pain scores preoperatively and at discharge were assessed. Intraoperative complications, urinary retention, postoperative nausea/vomiting, hospital transfers, and 90-day complications (reoperations, readmissions, and emergency department visits) were recorded.

Statistical Analysis
All statistics were evaluated using SPSS 26.0 (IBM, Chicago, IL). Descriptive statistics were performed for each of the variables listed above. The Shapiro-Wilk test was used to evaluate the day-of-surgery times and evaluate their distribution. They were found not to be normally distributed (operative time [$p < 0.001$], time until postoperative ambulation [$p = 0.034$], total postoperative facility duration [$p < 0.001$], and total facility duration [$p < 0.001$]); thus, median times and interquartile ranges (IQR) were used. Means and standard deviations were used for all other variables. Significance was set at $p < 0.05$.

RESULTS

There were 1,025 patients who had THA during the study period, sixty-nine (6.7%) of which were 65 years of age or older at the time of surgery and were included in this study. Table 1 lists demographic and preoperative patient information. Patients averaged 2.1 ± 1.5 medical comorbidities, with the most common being hypertension (38, 55%) and most (68, 99%) having an ASA classification of II or III. Alcohol abuse (>3 drinks per day) was noted in 6 patients (9%) and a third of patients used tobacco.

Day of surgery and intraoperative variables are listed in Table 2. Seven different surgeons had patients included. The majority of patients had a direct anterior approach (64, 93%)

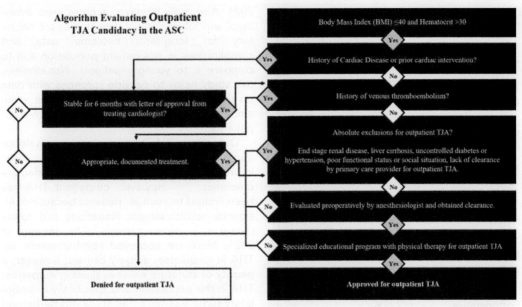

Fig. 1. Algorithm for the evaluation of outpatient total joint arthroplasty in an ambulatory surgery center.

Table 1	
Demographic and preoperative patient information	
Variables	**Results**
Age	67.9 ± 2.8
	≥70 years: 13 patients
	≥80: No patients
BMI	29.7 ± 5.8
Gender	35 Male
	34 Female
Comorbidities	2.1 ± 1.5/patient
	Hypertension: 38 (55%)
	Heart disease: 17 (25%)
	Mood disorder: 16 (23%)
	Diabetes: 9 (13%)
	Pulmonary disease (COPD, asthma, and so forth): 8 (12%)
Tobacco use	23 (33%)
Alcohol abuse	6 (9%)
ASA classification	I: 1 (1%)
	II: 51 (74%)
	III: 17 (25%)

Abbreviations: ASA, American society of anesthesiologists physical classification system; BMI, body mass index; COPD, chronic obstructive pulmonary disease.

determined by the operating surgeon and most had spinal anesthesia (65, 94%). Sixty-six patients (96%) met same-day discharge goals. Median facility duration was 8 hours and 45 minutes (8:45) (IQR 7:22, 10:06), with an operative time of 1:38 (IQR 1:29, 2:13). Two patients (3%) had next-day discharge from the facility, with one 72-year-old female having prolonged effects of spinal anesthesia leading to weakness and another 76-year-old male having urinary retention. Two other patients had postoperative urinary retention requiring discharge with a Foley catheter. Postoperative nausea that occurred in 15 patients resolved with medical management before discharge. One complication occurred in a 66-year-old female patient who experienced excessive blood loss during surgery and required hospital transfer for the transfusion of packed red blood cells. The patient was discharged the following day. The average VAS score was 3.9 ± 3.1 preoperatively and 1.0 ± 1.7 at discharge.

During the 90-day postoperative period, one patient required an emergency department visit for gastrointestinal issues caused by postoperative nonsteroidal anti-inflammatory drug (NSAID) regimen. No postoperative hospital admissions or reoperations were noted.

DISCUSSION

The results of this study demonstrate that outpatient THA can be safely performed in an ambulatory surgery center with predictable same-day

Table 2 Day of surgery and intraoperative variables	
Variables	**Results**
Total facility time	8:45 (IQR 7:22, 10:06)
Operative time	1:38 (IQR 1:29, 2:13)
Postoperative time to ambulation	3:31 (IQR 2:44. 4:39)
Postoperative facility time	4:50 (IQR 3:52, 6:35)
Approach	Direct Anterior: 64 (93%)
	Posterolateral: 5 (7%)
Anesthesia	Spinal: 65 (94%)
	General: 4 (6%)
EBL	340 ± 205 mL
Postoperative nausea/vomiting	15 (22%)
Postoperative urinary retention	2 (3%)
Ambulation distance	59 ± 36 ft
VAS (pain)	Facility arrival: 3.9 ± 3.1
	Facility discharge: 1.0 ± 1.7
Discharge Disposition	SDD: 66 (96%)
	NDD: 2 (3%)
	Prolonged spinal anesthesia/weakness (1), urinary retention (1)
	Transfer: 1 (1%)
	Acute blood loss anemia
Intraoperative and early postoperative complications	1 (1%), Acute blood loss anemia

Abbreviations: EBL, excessive blood loss; IQR, interquartile range; NDD, next day discharge; SDD, same day discharge; VAS, visual analog scale.

discharge and acceptable 90-day outcomes and complications in appropriately selected patients over the age of 65 years. The limitations of this study, however, cannot be overlooked. As a small retrospective, single-institution case series evaluating privately insured patients over the age of 65 years, selection bias is possible. Additionally, many Medicare-insured patients who may have been approriate candidates for THA at the ASC were unable to do so due to the restriction of reimbursement prior to January 2021. Also, only 90-day outcomes were evaluated, and future comparative studies are necessary for long-term outcome data and complications in this patient population and to compare it to younger patients. Nonetheless, this study helps to provide surgeons with data on the feasibility of same day discharge at an ambulatory surgery center in Medicare-aged patients.

Outpatient TJA is increasing in prevalence and is associated with decreased costs, improved patient satisfaction, and satisfactory outcomes.[4–6,19] However, outpatient THA has been limited to younger patients because of insurance reimbursement limitations and safety concerns in older patients.[12] In January of 2021, Medicare approved reimbursement for THA in ambulatory surgery centers; however, a paucity of literature exists evaluating outpatient THA in this population and specifically in ambulatory surgery centers. This study was performed to determine the safety of outpatient THA in ambulatory surgery centers in patients over the age of 65 years.

The definition of "outpatient" TJA has varied in the literature, ranging from same-day discharge from an ambulatory surgery center to 23- to 48-hour observation in a hospital.[15,16,20–22] McClatchy and colleagues.[20] examined the definition of "outpatient" TJA in the literature and found that less than 20% of outpatient THAs were performed in ambulatory surgery centers, with nearly 70% performed in a hospital with 23-hour observation. The discrepancy in the definition of "outpatient" leads to challenges when comparing studies. This discrepancy highlights the need for this study and others evaluating the safety of same-day discharge THA in ambulatory surgery centers.

Numerous algorithms have been published regarding patient selection for outpatient TJA; this study used those by Fournier and colleagues and Toy and colleagues[9,10] Age is a common variable in preoperative evaluation; however, this institution prefers a more nuanced, patient-specific approach that has shown acceptable outcomes in older patients.[23–28] Gronbeck and colleagues[15] developed an algorithm to identify patients requiring inpatient hospitalization (>2 days) after THA and found that age over 65 carried a weaker correlation with postoperative hospitalization than elevated body mass index (BMI), female gender, poor functional status, general anesthesia, procedure length, and medical comorbidities. Meneghini and colleagues created the Outpatient Arthroplasty Risk Assessment (OARA) score for the preoperative evaluation of outpatient TJA. They found that same-day and next-day discharge could be safely predicted without age being included as a risk factor for failure.[29] Instead of age, the OARA focuses on comorbidities, encapsulating multiple medical and social factors. The current study reinforces the need for broad preoperative patient evaluation before outpatient THA. Nearly all patients were ASA Class II or III, and many had multiple medical comorbidities; nevertheless, 96% were able to be discharged the same day (4.5 hours after surgery on average).

A steady increase in outpatient TJA was noted after the introduction of expedited postoperative protocols that lead to shorter hospitalizations and improved outcomes.[30–33] However, this trend has not been reflected in Medicare patients.[12,13,34] The few articles evaluating outpatient TJA in older patients largely rely on inpatient, national databases with mixed results. The lone, single-institution study evaluating outpatient THA in Medicare-aged patients highlighted a 93% same-day discharge rate from a hospital.[17] Another study using the PearlDiver database determined that outpatient THA (same-day or next-day discharge) was safe in appropriately selected patients.[35] Both studies highlighted similar complications between inpatient and outpatient cohorts.[17,35] However, studies using the American College of Surgeons National Surgery Quality Improvement Project (ACS-NSQIP) reported contrasting results.[14,36] Greenky and colleagues found that that less than 20% of patients older than 65 years were discharged on or before day 2 after THA, with only 1% being discharged the same day, and Sher and colleagues found that older patients were more likely to have delayed discharge and post-discharge complications.[14,36] Contrarily, a single-institution study in France by Pansard and colleagues[37] found patients who failed same-day discharge were on average younger (56.7 versus 61.4 years, p = 0.07) than those who were successfully discharged the same day as surgery. Although the lower same-day discharge percentages may be partially attributed to the decreased efficiency of hospitals compared with ambulatory surgery centers, this cannot account for the level of discrepancy in complication rates and discharge dispositions, calling into question NSQIP data.[38] In addition, after noting an 8% complication rate with same-day discharge after TJA compared to 2% after next-day discharge, Courtney and colleagues[39] recommended planned next-day discharge to avoid complications. Kraus and colleagues,[40] however, suggested that planned next-day discharge may be excessive, as 80% of their patients received no intervention overnight after TJA. Furthermore, a recent propensity score matched study with an average age of 66.5-years found that same day discharge TJA had no statistical difference in 90-day complications or readmissions compared to a traditional inpatient stay.[41] While outpatient THA may not be ideal for many elderly patients, this study found that with appropriate preoperative screening, THA can be safely performed in this patient population in ambulatory surgery centers with same-day discharge.

SUMMARY

In conclusion, older patients (≥65 years) undergoing outpatient THA in an ambulatory surgery center can safely undergo planned same-day discharge with acceptable perioperative and 90-day postoperative outcomes after appropriate preoperative evaluation, patient selection, and patient education. Additional studies are warranted to evaluate the results of this study and investigate the long-term safety of outpatient THA in this patient population.

CLINICS CARE POINTS

- Outpatient total joint arthroplasty is associated with decreased costs, improved patient satisfaction, and satisfactory outcomes; however, total hip arthroplasty in these settings has been limited to younger patients because of safety concerns in patients over the age of 65.

- Although age is a common prohibiting variable in same-day total hip arthroplasty, this study supports a more nuanced, patient-specific approach to achieve acceptable outcomes in older patients.

- Nearly all patients in this study were ASA Class II or III, and many had multiple medical comorbidities; nevertheless, 96% were able to be discharged the same day. Two patients required next day discharge, and one intraoperative complication required hospital transfer.

- Although outpatient THA is not ideal for many elderly patients, this study found that with appropriate preoperative screening, THA can be safely performed in this patient population in ambulatory surgery centers.

FUNDING

This research did not receive any specific grant from funding agencies in the public, commercial, or not-for-profit sectors.

ETHICAL REVIEW

This study was approved by the University of Tennessee Institutional Review Board (approval # 17–05344-XP) and informed patient consent was waived.

DISCLOSURES

Drs Z.A. Mosher, Calkins, Cope, and Pharr have no conflicts of interest to declare. Dr P.C. Toy reports personal fees from Innomed, Smith & Nephew, and Medtronic outside of the submitted work. Dr M.C. Ford declares personal fees from DePuy, A Johnson & Johnson Company, Osteoremedies, Medacta outside of the submitted work. Drs P.C. Toy and Ford are affiliated with free-standing ambulatory surgery centers.

REFERENCES

1. Sloan M, Sheth NP. Length of stay and inpatient mortality trends in primary and revision total joint arthroplasty in the United States, 2000-2014. J Orthop 2018;15:645–9.
2. Tarity TD, Swall MM. Current trends in discharge disposition and post-discharge care after total joint arthroplasty. Current Rev Musculoskelet Med 2017; 10:397–403.
3. Scully RD, Kappa JE, Melvin JS. "Outpatient"-same-calendar-day discharge hip and knee arthroplasty. J Am Acad Orthop Surg 2020;28:e900–99.
4. Bovonratwet P, Ondeck NT, Nelson SJ, et al. Comparison of outpatient vs inpatient total knee arthroplasty: an ACS-NSQIP analysis. J Arthroplasty 2017; 32:1773–8.
5. Pollock M, Somerville L, Firth A, et al. Outpatient total hip arthroplasty, total knee arthroplasty, and unicompartmental knee arthroplasty: a systematic review of the literature. JBJS Rev 2016;4. https://doi.org/10.2106/JBJS.RVW.16.00002. 01874474-201612000-00004.
6. Aynardi M, Post Z, Ong A, et al. Outpatient surgery as a means of cost reduction in total hip arthroplasty: a case-control study. HSS J 2014;10:252–5.
7. Kelly MP, Calkins TE, Culvern C, et al. Inpatient versus outpatient hip and knee arthroplasty: which has higher patient satisfaction? J Arthroplasty 2018; 33:3402–6.
8. Mundi R, Axelrod DE, Najafabadi BT, et al. Early discharge after total hip and knee arthroplasty-an observational cohort study evaluating safety in 330,000 patients. J Arthroplasty 2020;35:3482–7.e3.
9. Toy PC, Fournier MN, Throckmorton TW, et al. Low rates of adverse events following ambulatory outpatient total hip arthroplasty at a free-standing surgery center. J Arthroplasty 2018;33:46–50.
10. Fournier MN, Brolin TJ, Azar FM, et al. Identifying appropriate candidates for ambulatory outpatient shoulder arthroplasty: validation of a patient selection algorithm. J Shoulder Elbow Surg 2019;28:65–70.
11. Centers for Medicare and Medicaid Services. CY 2021 Medicare hospital outpatient prospective payment system and ambulatory surgical center payment system final rule (CMS-1736-FC). Available at: https://www.cms.gov/newsroom/fact-sheets/cy-2021-medicare-hospital-outpatient-prospective-payment-system-and-ambulatory surgical-center-0. Accessed January 24, 2021.
12. Lynch JC, Yayac M, Krueger CA, et al. Amount of CMS reduction in facility reimbursement following removal of total hip arthroplasty from the inpatient-only list far exceeds reduction in actual care cost. J Arthroplasty 2021;36(7):2276–80.
13. Centers for Medicare and Medicaid Services. Hospital Outpatient PPS. Web Baltimore, 255 MD: U.S. Centers for Medicare & Medicaid Services. Available at: 15 https://www.cms.gov/Medicare/Medic 256 are-Fee-for-Service Payment/Hospital-OutpatientPPS. Accessed September 28, 2020.
14. Greenky MR, Wang W, Ponzio DY, et al. Total hip arthroplasty and the Medicare inpatient-only list: an analysis of complications in Medicare-aged patients undergoing outpatient surgery. J Arthroplasty 2019; 34:1250–4.
15. Gronbeck CJ, Cote MP, Halawi MJ. Predicting inpatient status after total hip arthroplasty in Medicare-aged patients. J Arthroplasty 2019;34(2):249–54.
16. Goyal N, Chen AF, Padgett SE, et al. Otto aufranc award: a multicenter, randomized study of outpatient versus inpatient total hip arthroplasty. Clin Orthop Relat Res 2017;475:364–72.
17. Feder OI, Lygrisse K, Hutzler LH, et al. Outcomes of same-day discharge after total hip arthroplasty in the Medicare population. J Arthroplasty 2020;35:638–42.
18. Parvataneni HK, Ranawat AS, Ranawat CS. The use of local periarticular injections in the management of postoperative pain after total hip and knee replacement: a multimodal approach. Instr Course Lect 2007;56:125–31.
19. Bert JM, Hooper J, Moen S. Outpatient total joint arthroplasty. Curr Rev Musculoskelet Med 2017; 10(4):567–74.
20. McClatchy SG, Rider CM, Mihalko WM, et al. Defining outpatient hip and knee arthroplasties: a systematic review. J Am Acad Orthop Surg 2020.

https://doi.org/10.5435/JAAOS-D-19-00636. On-line ahead of print.16.

21. Shah RR, Cipparrone NE, Gordon AC, et al. Is it safe? Outpatient total joint arthroplasty with discharge to home at a freestanding ambulatory surgical center. Arthroplast Today 2018;4(4):484–7.

22. Jaibaji M, Volpin A, Haddad FS, et al. Is outpatient arthroplasty safe? A systematic review. J Arthroplasty 2020;35:1941–9.

23. Divo MJ, Martinez CH, Mannino DM. Ageing and the epidemiology of multimorbidity. Eur Respir J 2014;44:1055–68.

24. Fortin M, Bravo G, Hudon C, et al. Relationship between multimorbidity and health-related quality of life of patients in primary care. Qual Life Res 2006;15:83–91.

25. Stenholm S, Westerlund H, Head J, et al. Comorbidity and functional trajectories from midlife to old age: the health and retirement study. J Gerontol A Biol Sci Med Sci 2014;70:332–8.

26. Bayliss EA, Ellis JL, Steiner JF. Barriers to self-management and quality-of-life outcomes in seniors with multimorbidities. Ann Fam Med 2007; 5(5):395–402.

27. Ogino D, Kawaji H, Konttinen L, et al. Total hip replacement in patients eighty years of age and older. J Bone Joint Surg Am 2008;90:1884–90.

28. Jones CA, Voaklander DC, Johnston DWC, et al. the effect of age on pain, function, and quality of life after total hip and knee arthroplasty. Arch Intern Med 2001;161:454–60.

29. Meneghini RM, Ziemba-Davis M, Ishmael MK, et al. Safe selection of outpatient joint arthroplasty patients with medical risk stratification: the "Outpatient Arthroplasty Risk Assessment Score". J Arthroplasty 2017;32:2325–31.

30. Bertin KC. Minimally invasive outpatient total hip arthroplasty: a financial analysis. Clin Orthop Relat Res 2005;435:154–63.

31. Berger RA, Jacobs JJ, Meneghini RM, et al. Rapid rehabilitation and recovery with minimally invasive total hip arthroplasty. Clin Orthop Relat 2004;429: 230–47.

32. Backstein D, Thiagarajah S, Halawi MJ, et al. Outpatient total knee arthroplasty-the new reality and how can it be achieved? J Arthroplasty 2018; 33:3595–8.

33. Buller LT, Hubbard TA, Ziemba-Davis M, et al. Safety of same and next day discharge following revision hip and knee arthroplasty using modern perioperative protocols. J Arthroplasty 2021;36:30–6.

34. Halawi MJ, Stone AD, Gronbeck C, et al. Medicare coverage is an independent predictor of prolonged hospitalization after primary total joint arthroplasty. Arthroplast Today 2019;5:489–92.

35. Arshi A, Leong NL, Wang C, et al. Outpatient total hip arthroplasty in the United States: a population-based comparative analysis of complication rates. J Am Acad Orthop Surg 2019;27:61–7.

36. Sher A, Keswani A, Yao DH, et al. Predictors of same day discharge in primary total joint arthroplasty patients and risk factors for post325 discharge complications. J Arthroplasty 2017;32:150–6.e1.

37. Pansard E, Klouche S, Bauer T, et al. Can primary total hip arthroplasty be performed in an outpatient setting? Prospective feasibility and safety study in 321 patients in a day-surgery unit. Orthop Traumatol Surg Res 2020;106(3):551–5.

38. Kadhim M, Gans I, Baldwin K, et al. Do surgical times and efficiency differ between inpatient and ambulatory surgery centers that are both hospital owned? J Pediatr Orthop 2016;36:423–8.

39. Courtney PM, Froimson MI, Meneghini RM, et al. Can total knee arthroplasty be performed safely as an outpatient in the Medicare population? J Arthroplasty 2018;33:S28–31.

40. Kraus KR, Buller LT, Caccavallo PP, et al. Is there benefit in keeping early discharge patients overnight after total joint arthroplasty? J Arthroplasty 2021;36:24–9.

41. Jenny JY, Gisonni V. Complications of total hip or knee arthroplasty are not significantly more common after ambulatory surgery than after in-patient surgery and enhanced recovery: a case-control study with propensity-score matching. Orthop Traumatol Surg Res 2022;108(2):103206.

Knee and Hip Reconstruction

Management of Intraoperative Acetabular Fractures During Total Hip Arthroplasty

Taylor P. Stauffer, BS[a,b,*], Kevin F. Purcell, MD, MPH, MS[c],
Christian Pean, MD, MS[c], Malcolm DeBaun, MD[c],
Michael Bolognesi, MD[c], Sean Ryan, MD[c],
Danielle Chun, MD[c], Thorsten Seyler, MD, PhD[c]

KEYWORDS

- Total hip arthroplasty • Periprosthetic fracture • Hip fracture

KEY POINTS

- Intraoperative acetabular fracture during total hip arthroplasty (THA) is rare; however, it can be occult and can lead to severe complications if not addressed.
- There are several risk factors associated with intraoperative fracture, including cup geometry, patient factors, and use of press-fit components, among others.
- Acute fractures generally require attention with plating, whereas chronic acetabular fractures may be approached with distraction, a Burch-Schneider cage, or a custom implant.
- Consider missed intraoperative acetabular fracture with persistent groin pain after THA.

INTRODUCTION

Periprosthetic fractures of the acetabulum during total hip arthroplasty (THA) are rare complications that can profoundly affect postoperative outcomes, affecting stability, survival, and migration of acetabular components. Occult intraoperative periprosthetic acetabular fractures, although infrequently reported, are associated with persistent pain and diminished implant survival after THA and can present weeks postsurgery as persistent groin pain.[1,2]

The incidence of overt intraoperative femoral fractures during THA has been reported to range from 0.1% to 1% and up to 5% for cemented and uncemented primary THA, with a projected increase due to the growing demand for THA and decrease in mortality index.[3–11] However, intraoperative acetabular fractures have received comparatively less attention, possibly due to their relative rarity or difficulty in detection. Existing literature reports a prevalence as low as 0.4% during uncemented cup fixation, increasing to 0.7% for all THAs.[12,13]

Multiple factors contribute to the risk of acetabular fractures during the THA procedure, including iatrogenic factors such as underreaming, overreaming, and implant impaction during cementless component fixation.[12,14–16] Cadaveric studies have shown that oversized component insertion can lead to acetabular fractures; this is less common if line-to-line reaming is performed.[17] Conversely, smaller cups less than 50 mm have also been shown to pose a higher risk for intraoperative fracture.[18–20] Pathologic factors encompass osteoporosis, osteolysis, infection, dysplasia, cancer, diabetes mellitus, rheumatoid arthritis, and Paget disease.[13,16,21–23] Patients undergoing revision THA face a higher

[a] School of Medicine, Duke University, Durham, NC, USA; [b] Duke University Hospital, 40 Duke Medicine Circle, Durham, NC 27710, USA; [c] Division of Orthopedic Surgery, Duke University, Durham, NC, USA
* Corresponding author. Duke University Hospital, 40 Duke Medicine Circle, Durham, NC 27710.
E-mail address: Taylor.stauffer@duke.edu

Orthop Clin N Am 55 (2024) 9–17
https://doi.org/10.1016/j.ocl.2023.06.009
0030-5898/24/© 2023 Elsevier Inc. All rights reserved.

likelihood of intraoperative acetabular fracture compared with primary THA due to challenging surgical factors, such as the removal of well-fixed acetabular components that require excessive force for extraction.[24] Preventative measures are largely patient-specific encompassing line-to-line reaming, preoperative optimization of patient health, cementless versus cemented acetabular component insertion, and appropriate implant sizing.

Cup geometry seems to play an important role as well, especially with the popularity of cementless sockets. Cementless acetabular components can be inserted with line-to-line reaming or by underreaming the acetabulum with press-fit impaction.[25] Components can be elliptical with a peripheral flare, hemispheric, or peripheral self-locking, with a rim that is 1.8 mm larger than the cup diameter. Prior research has demonstrated that the impaction of elliptical monoblock cementless cups is more likely to result in fracture than hemispherical modular cementless cup.[1,12,17,26] Moreover, in a study of 406 patients undergoing THA, Hasegawa and colleagues[27] reported an increased risk of occult acetabular fracture with press-fit impaction of peripheral self-locking cups compared with hemispheric cups. Fractures were most frequently found on the superolateral wall with postoperative computed tomography (CT) scans. The risk of fracture is further heightened in patients with poor bone stock, sclerotic bone, and smaller pelvic footprints.[1]

Management of acetabular fractures depends on an acute or chronic presentation. As will be discussed later in the article, acute fractures generally require attention with plating, whereas chronic acetabular fractures can be approached with distraction, a Burch-Schneider cage, or a custom implant.[28,29] It is also important to note that THA itself is often a treatment of acute acetabular fractures, especially in the elderly population.[30,31]

Currently, there is no universally accepted treatment algorithm for intraoperative acetabular fractures, and literature on this topic remains scarce. Given the rarity of these fractures and their complex treatment, our narrative review aims to provide a comprehensive overview of the current literature on intraoperative acetabular fractures during THA and our institutional perioperative management. By discussing treatment options and postoperative considerations, we seek to offer guidance to surgeons facing these intricate challenges, helping them achieve optimal patient outcomes, hip stability, and proper management.

CLASSIFICATION AND MANAGEMENT OF INTRAOPERATIVE ACETABULAR FRACTURES

Classification

Navigating the complexities of intraoperative acetabular fractures and assessing stability are crucial in preventing aseptic loosening and poor outcomes. In 1996, Peterson and Lewallen introduced a classification system for acetabular fractures after THA, which has since evolved through various adaptations: type 1: clinical and radiographic stability of the acetabular component; type 2: the acetabular component was deemed unstable.[13] Laflamme and colleagues[32] added the type 3 acetabular fracture, which is a missed intraoperative acetabular fracture noticed on postoperative radiographs. Perhaps the most comprehensive and widely used systems today are the 1995 Vancouver system and the 2003 Paprosky and Della Valle classification, which take multiple factors into account and serve as a foundation for fracture management.[33,34] Davidson and colleagues[35] further simplified the Paprosky and Della Valle system detailing the following 3 fracture types: I: nondisplaced and not compromising stability of reconstruction, II: nondisplaced that may compromise stability of reconstruction; III: displaced. More recently, a classification proposal by Pascarella and colleagues[10] in 2019 incorporates fracture timing. Despite limited therapeutic use and complexity, it is worth noting the 2014 unified classification system, which assesses stability, location, and associated fracture features (Table 1).[36]

Conservative Management

Per the Paprosky and Della Valle classification system, type 1 fractures can typically be treated without any type of augmentation. To ensure the best outcomes, arthroplasty surgeons must be well versed in the geometry of the acetabular component and adhere to appropriate reaming protocols. It is important to note that many of type I fractures are often not recognized in the intraoperative setting. Interestingly, Haidukewych and colleagues[12] reported a significant increase in intraoperative acetabular fractures when using an acetabular component with an elliptical flare.

Intraoperative acetabular fractures during THA are rather rare and can possibly go unnoticed for weeks.[32] Generally, intraoperative acetabular fractures can be managed without any supplemental plating or screw augmentation. Intraoperative acetabular fractures can occur during acetabular reaming, component impaction, or hip dislocation. It is important to frequently inspect the acetabulum, especially

Table 1 Adaptation of the evolution of periprosthetic acetabular fracture classification systems			
Classification System	**Factors**	**Types**	**Subtypes**
Vancouver (1995)	*Location, stability, configuration*	*Type A: proximal metaphyseal* *Type B: diaphyseal* *Type C: distal fractures beyond longest revision stem, can include distal metaphysis*	*Subtype 1: simple cortical perforation* *Subtype 2: nondisplaced linear crack* *Subtype 2: displaced or unstable*
Peterson and Lewellen (1996)	*Stability, pain*	*Type 1: acetabular component clinically and radiographically stable. Minimal pain with hip motion* *Type 2: unstable acetabular component. Painful hip motion*	—
LaFlamme (1998)	*Stability*	*Same as Peterson and Lewellen, but with the following* *Type 3: missed intraoperative acetabular fracture seen on postoperative radiographs*	—
Paprosky and Della Valle (2003)	*Timing, method, stability*	*Type1: intraoperative during component insertion* *Type 2: intraoperative during removal* *Type 3: traumatic* *Type 4: spontaneous* *Type 5: pelvic discontinuity*	*1A: recognized, stable, nondisplaced* *1B: recognized, unstable, displaced* *1C: not recognized* *2A: <50% bone loss* *2B: >50% bone loss* *3A: stable component* *3B: unstable component* *4A: <50% bone loss* *4B: >50% bone loss* *5A: <50% bone loss* *5B: >50% bone loss* *5C: associated with radiation*
United Classification System (UCS) (2014)	*Stability, location, anatomic features*	*A: apophyseal or extraarticular/ periarticular* *B: bed of implant or around implant* *C: distant to implant* *D: dividing the bone between 2 implants* *E: each of 2 bones supporting 1 arthroplasty* *F: facing and articulating with a hemiarthroplasty*	*B1: stable prosthesis, good bone* *B2: loose prosthesis, good bone* *B2: loose prosthesis, bad bone* *Specific to hip:* *IV.6: acetabulum/pelvis* *IV.3: femur, proximal*

(continued on next page)

Table 1 (continued)			
Classification System	**Factors**	**Types**	**Subtypes**
Pascarella (2019)	*Timing, stability*	Type 1: *intraoperative* Type 2: *postoperative/ traumatic*	1A: *stable prosthesis* 1B: *unstable prosthesis* 2A: *stable prosthesis* 2B: *unstable prosthesis* 2C: *unstable prosthesis, mobilized before trauma*

the anterior/posterior wall during each step to ensure there are no visible fracture lines or eccentrically reaming. Moreover, intraoperative acetabular fracture should also be suspected when the cup sits more medial than expected or the surgeon is not achieving the expected press-fit fixation. The arthroplasty surgeon should consider occult acetabular fracture in patients with persistent groin pain after THA. Because these fractures may not be visualized on intra- and postoperative radiographs, they warrant CT pelvis scan for further evaluation.[2]

Li and colleagues and Haidukewych and colleagues have published the largest series to date of intraoperative acetabular fractures.[12,37] In the study by Haidukewych and colleagues, 17 of 21 patients were managed without any supplemental plating due to stability of the acetabular component. In the remaining 4 patients, another acetabular component was used that allowed for multiple screws to be placed through the acetabular component. Li and colleagues[37] reported that 20 out of 24 of their patients underwent multiscrew fixation of the acetabular component, and the remaining 4 did not warrant any screw augmentation. Thus, it is important that arthroplasty surgeons are familiar with the pelvic anatomy and safe zone for screw placement, and it remains a key pillar in the treatment of acetabular fractures.

At our institution, on identifying an intraoperative fracture, we immediately halt reaming and instrumentation to visually inspect the entirety of the acetabulum. The focus is on preventing further fracture propagation and identifying noncontiguous fracture lines. We also assess the integrity of the medial wall to ensure that the acetabular component can be safely impacted without compromising the medial wall. The integrity of the posterior column is also assessed to discern if a traumatologist should be consulted to assist with plating of the posterior column (Case 1). Intraoperative fractures of the posterior acetabular column portend worse outcomes and higher failure rates.[32] If stability is deemed to be adequate for a primary cementless acetabular component, then the acetabular component is augmented with

screw fixation. However, it would be advisable to add bone graft from the femoral head or sequential reaming into the noted defect. The investigators believe it is prudent to augment acetabular fixation with at least 3 screws through the acetabular shell, but this is surgeon dependent.

Plating of the Anterior or Posterior Column

A critical challenge in stabilizing intraoperative acetabular fractures is determining whether fracture fixation can be achieved using the same approach used for THA. For instance, with a direct anterior or anterior-based muscle-sparing approach, it becomes unfeasible to plate the posterior column in the event of a transverse, posterior column, or posterior wall fracture. Thus, an additional approach would be required to stabilize these areas of the pelvis with plate and screws. Furthermore, when dealing with an intraoperative acetabular fracture involving the anterior column, a modified Stoppa and ilioinguinal approach may be needed if a posterior- or lateral-based approach is being used for THA. In such cases, it would be prudent for the arthroplasty surgeon to consult with an orthopedic traumatologist for assistance in managing these complexities.

At our institution, most of the THAs, particularly conversion THAs, are performed through a posterior-based approach. If posterior column plating is warranted, our orthopedic traumatologist partners are often consulted to assist with single or dual-plate fixation to the posterior column. In addition, they assess the need for an anterior column screw. Failure of the acetabular component after intraoperative acetabular fractures is secondary to instability of the posterior column.[32] Plating of the posterior column is crucial, especially in the acute setting, for successful outcomes and osteointegration of the acetabular component when significant posterior column involvement is present. An anterior intrapelvic buttress plate may be placed to lateralize the acetabulum if there is significant medialization of the femoral head secondary to a destabilizing fracture involving the quadrilateral surface.

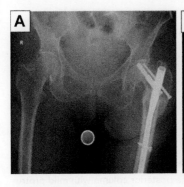
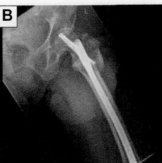

Fig. 1. (A) Anteroposterior (AP) and (B) lateral radiographs of a left hip that underwent previous cephalomedullary nailing for left hip fracture. Notice the reverse Z-phenomenon (inferior lag screw migrated medially cutting through the femoral head and the superior lag screw).

Acetabular Distraction

It is important to assess the stability of the fracture if a fracture line is noticed along the medial wall or acetabular roof. There is the chance that an acetabular component may not be able to obtain adequate press fit fixation with a primary acetabular component. A technique that we commonly use at our institution (Case 1) is acetabular distraction. If press-fit fixation is not occurring, we assess the stability of the acetabulum to sustain acetabular distraction. The acetabulum is reamed until we have engagement of the anterosuperior and posteroinferior regions of the acetabulum at the periphery and not medializing during this process. We ream roughly 3 to 5 mm less than the impacted cup. Subsequently, several screws are placed through a revision acetabular component to augment fixation. It would be prudent for the arthroplasty surgeon to place bone graft from acetabular reaming into the fracture lines and at the center of the acetabulum.

Acetabular Roof Reinforcement Plate

Resch and colleagues and Krappinger have described the use of an acetabular roof reinforcement plate (Depuy Synthes, Battlach, Switzerland) for management of geriatric acetabular fractures.[31,38] This construct consists of an inner and outer diameter that fits within the acetabulum

and an upper fin on the top side of the ring, which has several screw holes to place 3.5-mm screws. This plate provides robust support for acetabular component placement. Although Resch and colleagues' technique was not specifically designed for intraoperative acetabular fractures, it can be used as an option, depending on the severity of the fracture. The key advantage of this plate is that it allows patients to weight-bear immediately after surgery, eliminating the need for restrictions of weight-bearing status. However, using this acetabular roof reinforcement plate through an anterior-based approach may prove challenging.

CASE

Case 1

Patient 1 is an 83-year-old woman with multiple medical comorbidities that previously sustained a left pertrochanteric fracture after a fall from standing. She underwent cephalomedullary nailing to stabilize her left hip. She was previously a community ambulator using a cane for assistance with mobilization. During her postoperative course, she sustained screw cutout of the left hip cephalomedullary nailing (Fig. 1) with concomitant progression of left hip osteoarthritis.

She underwent a left conversion THA for the progression of osteoarthritis and screw cutout of the cephalomedullary nail. This conversion

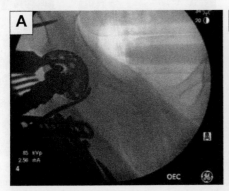
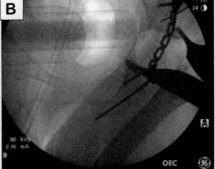

Fig. 2. Intraoperative fluoroscopic images demonstrating (A) fracture of the posterior column during reaming. (B) The posterior column was plated for additional stability.

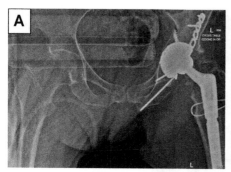
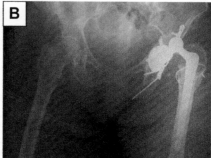

Fig. 3. (A) Immediate postoperative radiographs demonstrating plating of the posterior column with mild protrusion of the acetabular component. (B) The patient sustained a posterosuperior dislocation POD 2. Patient was managed with closed reduction. Due to persistent instability, CT pelvis was ordered to assess acetabular component orientation.

was performed through a Kocher-Langenbeck approach. Intraoperatively it was noted she had a greater trochanter deformity and a shallow acetabulum. The reaming of the acetabulum led to an acetabular fracture that was deemed to be stable (Fig. 2). Impaction of the acetabular component led to propagation of fracture along the anterior and posterior columns. At this point, the posterior column was exposed in standard fashion with identification of the sciatic nerve, before plate application. A single 3.5-mm pelvic reconstruction plate was contoured to the acetabulum, and this was thought to provide adequate stability of the posterior column.

She sustained 2 posterosuperior dislocations (Fig. 3) within 2 weeks of her conversion THA. She was managed with closed reduction under sedation initially. A pelvic CT scan was obtained secondary to acute instability and demonstrated retroversion of the acetabular component (Fig. 4). The version of the femoral component was deemed to be in good alignment. As previously noted, after intraoperative acetabular fracture during THA there is a likelihood that the acetabular components can fall into retroversion.

The decision was made to revise her acetabular component. She was brought to the operating room within 3 weeks of her index conversion THA for her left revision THA. Intraoperatively, it was noted the acetabular component was mildly retroverted, and there was posterior instability. The acetabular components were removed, and a defect in the medial wall was noted. After intraoperative assessment, it was decided additional fixation with an anterior column screw was not necessary. Acetabular reaming was undertaken, and a 57-mm (mm) reamer was last used. Bone graft was placed in the medial defect to assist with developing callus along the previous fracture

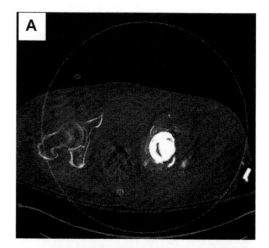
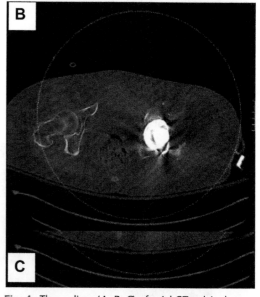

Fig. 4. Three slices (A, B, C) of axial CT pelvis demonstrating retroversion of the acetabular component; likely the cause of her postoperative instability contributing to the posterosuperior dislocation.

site. Subsequently, a Redapt (Smith and Nephew, Memphis, TN, USA) 60-mm multihole dual mobility acetabular component was inserted (**Fig. 5**). Underreaming by 3 mm allowed for a press fit. Several screws were inserted in the sciatic buttress to augment the fixation. She was kept toe-touch weight-bearing for 6 weeks, and her weight-bearing status subsequently advanced to weight-bearing as tolerated. At her 7-month visit, she is pain free, ambulating without difficulty, and has not sustained any additional dislocations or other postoperative complications.

POSTOPERATIVE PRECAUTIONS
Weight-Bearing Status
Weight-bearing as tolerated (WBAT) is the standard protocol after primary THA. However, the weight-bearing status after an intraoperative fracture during THA is fracture-, treatment-, and surgeon-dependent. Typically, at our institution, we will start patients with foot-flat weight-bearing for 3 to 4 weeks and then advance to weight-bearing as tolerated. However, there are rare instances if acetabular fixation is thought to be stable that we will allow the patient to be WBAT immediately after surgery.

Hip Precautions
At our institution, patients are placed on posterior hip precautions if they sustained an intraoperative acetabular fracture during a posterior-based approach for THA and anterior precautions if there was an acetabular fracture during an anterior-based approach. It is important to check range of motion and stability after plating of the posterior column and placement of acetabular cup/stem after sustaining an intraoperative acetabular fracture. It is important to visualize acetabular and femoral version after sustaining a fracture. There is always the potential that component can have either too much retroversion or too much anteversion and should be rectified before leaving the operating room.

Special Considerations
Deep vein thrombosis prophylaxis
Deep vein thrombosis (DVT) prophylaxis for pelvis/acetabular fractures is not the same as primary THA. At our institution, the current DVT prophylaxis protocol for primary THA is aspirin 81 mg twice daily.[39] If a patient is on an anticoagulant for a preexisting DVT, cardiovascular disease, and so on, we cease their anticoagulant medication and restart it 48 hours after THA. In the interim, they are provided low-molecular-weight heparin (Lovenox) until restarting their anticoagulant medication.

However, the DVT prophylaxis protocol is different for pelvis/acetabular fractures. Lovenox, 30 mg, twice daily is used after open

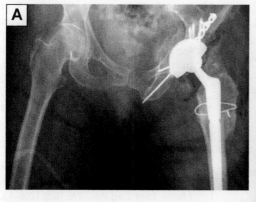
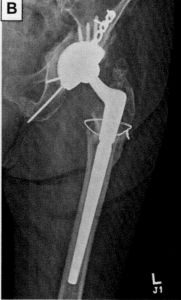

Fig. 5. (A) Immediate postoperative radiographs after revision of the acetabular component. (B) Six-month postoperative AP left hip radiograph demonstrating healing bridged callus along the posterior column and maintained alignment of the acetabular component.

reduction internal fixation for the fracture. This same DVT prophylaxis is used for an intraoperative pelvis/acetabular fracture during THA. This situation is no longer treated as a standard primary THA. However, in the recent PREVENT CLOT study it was rendered that aspirin was noninferior to Lovenox in preventing death, 90-day readmissions, and for DVT prophylaxis.[40]

SUMMARY

Intraoperative acetabular fracture, although rare, can lead to severe complications if not properly addressed. It is imperative for arthroplasty surgeons to possess a thorough understanding of how to identify and manage these injuries. Collaborating with an orthopedic traumatologist for assistance with plating the anterior or posterior column, if necessary, can be invaluable. Management options encompass conservative management, revision style acetabular component, screw/plating of anterior/posterior column, and the use of a larger cup with multiple screw augmentation options.

CLINICS CARE POINTS

- Continually inspect acetabulum during THA especially when reaming and cup impaction.
- Consider missed intraoperative acetabular fracture with persistent groin pain after THA.
- After intraoperative acetabular fracture discern if cup augmentation or plating of anterior/posterior column is warranted.
- Surgeon should familiarize himself/herself with geometry of cup and the reaming protocol.
- Consider patient's comorbidities when prescribing DVT prophylaxis.

DISCLOSURE

M. DeBaun Summit Surgical Corp: education. Smith and Nephew: food and beverage. C. Pean Stryker, OsteoCentric: food and beverage. S. Ryan Smith and Nephew, Encore Medical, DePuy Synthes, Bioventus: travel and lodging. M. Bolognesi Zimmer Biomet: Royalty, License, food and beverage, Smith and Nephew: Royalty, License, Total Joint Orthopaedics: Royalty, License. Ethicon: Consulting. Heron Therapeutics: Consulting. T. Seyler: Smith and Nephew: Consulting, faculty or speaker at venue. All other authors have nothing to disclose. T Stauffer: Eugene A. Stead Fellowship Fund.

REFERENCES

1. Sharkey PF, Hozack WJ, Callaghan JJ, et al. Acetabular fracture associated with cementless acetabular component insertion: a report of 13 cases. J Arthroplasty 1999;14(4):426–31.
2. Dammerer D, Putzer D, Glodny B, et al. Occult intra-operative periprosthetic fractures of the acetabulum may affect implant survival. Int Orthop 2019;43(7):1583–90.
3. Kavanagh BF. Femoral fractures associated with total hip arthroplasty. Orthop Clin North Am 1992; 23(2):249–57.
4. Jensen JS, Retpen JB. Failures with the Judet non-cemented total hip. Acta Orthop Scand 1987;58(1): 23–6.
5. Berry DJ. Epidemiology: hip and knee. Orthop Clin North Am 1999;30(2):183–90.
6. Mayle RE, Della Valle CJ. Intra-operative fractures during THA: see it before it sees us. J Bone Joint Surg Br 2012;94(11 Suppl A):26–31.
7. Schwartz JT Jr, Mayer JG, Engh CA. Femoral fracture during non-cemented total hip arthroplasty. J Bone Joint Surg Am 1989;71(8):1135–42.
8. Taylor MM, Meyers MH, Harvey JP Jr. Intraoperative femur fractures during total hip replacement. Clin Orthop Relat Res 1978;(137):96–103.
9. Ricioli W Jr, Queiroz MC, Guimarães RP, et al. Prevalence and risk factors for intra-operative periprosthetic fractures in one thousand eight hundred and seventy two patients undergoing total hip arthroplasty: a cross-sectional study. Int Orthop 2015; 39(10):1939–43.
10. Pascarella R, Sangiovanni P, Cerbasi S, et al. Periprosthetic acetabular fractures: a new classification proposal. Injury 2018;49(Suppl 3):S65–73.
11. Kurtz S, Ong K, Lau E, et al. Projections of primary and revision hip and knee arthroplasty in the United States from 2005 to 2030. J Bone Joint Surg Am 2007;89(4):780–5.
12. Haidukewych GJ, Jacofsky DJ, Hanssen AD, et al. Intraoperative fractures of the acetabulum during primary total hip arthroplasty. J Bone Joint Surg Am 2006;88(9):1952–6.
13. Peterson CA, Lewallen DG. Periprosthetic fracture of the acetabulum after total hip arthroplasty. J Bone Joint Surg Am 1996;78(8):1206–13.
14. Benazzo F, Formagnana M, Bargagliotti M, et al. Periprosthetic acetabular fractures. Int Orthop 2015;39(10):1959–63.
15. Ivanova S, Vuillemin N, Hapa O, et al. Revision of a failed primary total hip arthroplasty following excessive reaming with a medial cup protrusion. Medicina (Kaunas) 2022;58(9). https://doi.org/10.3390/medicina58091254.
16. Takigami I, Ito Y, Mizoguchi T, et al. Pelvic discontinuity caused by acetabular overreaming during

primary total hip arthroplasty. Case Rep Orthop 2011;2011:939202.

17. Kim YS, Callaghan JJ, Ahn PB, et al. Fracture of the acetabulum during insertion of an oversized hemispherical component. J Bone Joint Surg Am 1995; 77(1):111–7.

18. Dorr LD, Faugere MC, Mackel AM, et al. Structural and cellular assessment of bone quality of proximal femur. Bone 1993;14(3):231–42.

19. Lamb JN, Matharu GS, Redmond A, et al. Risk factors for intraoperative periprosthetic femoral fractures during primary total hip arthroplasty. an analysis from the national joint registry for England and wales and the isle of man. J Arthroplasty 2019;34(12):3065–73.e1.

20. Brown JM, Borchard KS, Robbins CE, et al. Management and prevention of intraoperative acetabular fracture in primary total hip arthroplasty. Am J Orthop (Belle Mead NJ) 2017;46(5):232–7.

21. McGrory BJ. Periprosthetic fracture of the acetabulum during total hip arthroplasty in a patient with Paget's disease. Am J Orthop (Belle Mead NJ) 1999;28(4):248–50.

22. Zwartelé RE, Witjes S, Doets HC, et al. Cementless total hip arthroplasty in rheumatoid arthritis: a systematic review of the literature. Arch Orthop Trauma Surg 2012;132(4):535–46.

23. Chatoo M, Parfitt J, Pearse MF. Periprosthetic acetabular fracture associated with extensive osteolysis. J Arthroplasty 1998;13(7):843–5.

24. Chitre A, Wynn Jones H, Shah N, et al. Complications of total hip arthroplasty: periprosthetic fractures of the acetabulum. Curr Rev Musculoskelet Med 2013;6(4):357–63.

25. García-Rey E, García-Cimbrelo E, Cruz-Pardos A. Cup press fit in uncemented THA depends on sex, acetabular shape, and surgical technique. Clin Orthop Relat Res 2012;470(11):3014–23.

26. Yun HH, Cheon SH, Im JT, et al. Periprosthetic occult acetabular fracture: an unknown side effect of press-fit techniques in primary cementless total hip arthroplasty. Eur J Orthop Surg Traumatol 2021;31(7):1411–9.

27. Hasegawa K, Kabata T, Kajino Y, et al. Periprosthetic occult fractures of the acetabulum occur frequently during primary THA. Clin Orthop Relat Res 2017;475(2):484–94.

28. Liaw F, Govilkar S, Banks D, et al. Primary total hip replacement using Burch-Schneider cages for acetabular fractures. Hip Int 2022;32(3):401–6.

29. Tidermark J, Blomfeldt R, Ponzer S, et al. Primary total hip arthroplasty with a Burch-Schneider antiprotrusion cage and autologous bone grafting for acetabular fractures in elderly patients. J Orthop Trauma 2003;17(3):193–7.

30. Schnaser E, Scarcella NR, Vallier HA. Acetabular fractures converted to total hip arthroplasties in the elderly: how does function compare to primary total hip arthroplasty? J Orthop Trauma 2014; 28(12):694–9.

31. Resch H, Krappinger D, Moroder P, et al. Treatment of acetabular fractures in older patients-introduction of a new implant for primary total hip arthroplasty. Arch Orthop Trauma Surg 2017; 137(4):549–56.

32. Laflamme GY, Belzile EL, Fernandes JC, et al. Periprosthetic fractures of the acetabulum during cup insertion: posterior column stability is crucial. J Arthroplasty 2015;30(2):265–9.

33. Della Valle CJ, Momberger NG, Paprosky WG. Periprosthetic fractures of the acetabulum associated with a total hip arthroplasty. Instr Course Lect 2003;52:281–90.

34. Masri BA, Meek RMD, Duncan CP. Periprosthetic Fractures evaluation and treatment. Clin Orthop Relat Res 2004;420:80–95.

35. Davidson D, Pike J, Garbuz D, et al. Intraoperative periprosthetic fractures during total hip arthroplasty. Evaluation and management. J Bone Joint Surg Am 2008;90(9):2000–12.

36. Duncan CP, Haddad FS. The unified classification system (UCS): improving our understanding of periprosthetic fractures. The Bone & Joint Journal 2014;96-B(6):713–6.

37. Li Y-H, Yu T, Shao W, et al. Distal locked versus unlocked intramedullary nailing for stable intertrochanteric fractures, a systematic review and meta-analysis. BMC Muscoskel Disord 2020;21(1): 461.

38. Krappinger D, Resch H, Lindtner RA, et al. The acetabular roof reinforcement plate for the treatment of displaced acetabular fractures in the elderly: results in 59 patients. Arch Orthop Trauma Surg 2022;142(8):1835–45.

39. Haykal T, Kheiri B, Zayed Y, et al. Aspirin for venous thromboembolism prophylaxis after hip or knee arthroplasty: an updated meta-analysis of randomized controlled trials. J Orthop 2019; 16(4):294–302.

40. O'Toole RV, Stein DM, Frey KP, et al. PREVENTion of CLots in Orthopaedic Trauma (PREVENT CLOT): a randomised pragmatic trial protocol comparing aspirin versus low-molecular-weight heparin for blood clot prevention in orthopaedic trauma patients. BMJ Open 2021;11(3):e041845.

Treatment of Intraoperative Trochanteric Fractures During Primary and Revision Total Hip Arthroplasty

Akram A. Habibi, MD, Ran Schwarzkopf, MD, MSc*

KEYWORDS

- Trochanteric fractures • Total hip arthroplasty • Greater trochanter • Complications • Cables
- Claw plates

KEY POINTS

- Although trochanteric fractures are infrequent, surgeons should remain particularly vigilant for intraoperative trochanteric fractures during uncemented primary and revision total hip arthroplasty.
- Surgeons should have high suspicion of fracture when there is a loss of resistance or acoustic changes during impaction of the broach or stem.
- Patient activity level, bone mineral density, and fracture morphology should be used to assist in determining appropriate fixation strategies.
- Treatment options include conservative management, cable or wire fixation, cable grip fixation, or plate fixation.
- Patients should have limited weight-bearing, preferably with assistive device, and no active abduction for 6 weeks postoperatively.

INTRODUCTION

Intraoperative trochanteric fractures are serious complications that can arise during primary and revision total hip arthroplasty (THA). There are a variety of factors that can lead to these fractures, including surgical technique, bone quality, and implant design. A study by Berry and colleagues[1] examined intraoperative periprosthetic fractures during THA and found that cemented primary THA had a rate of 0.3% intraoperative fractures, whereas uncemented primary THA had a rate of 5.4%. The same study also found that in revision THA, there was a rate of 3.6% intraoperative femoral fractures for cemented revisions compared with 20.9% in uncemented revision. In addition to surgical technique, patient factors also have an effect on the risk of

intraoperative trochanteric fractures. Female patients and older age have an increased risk of intraoperative fracture during THA owing to diminished bone mineral density in the setting of osteoporosis.[2]

Although trochanteric fractures can occur at any time during a THA, certain portions of the procedure are at increased risk of causing this complication. Abdel and colleagues[2] examined 132 intraoperative trochanteric fractures in patients with primary THA and found that 83.7% of trochanteric fractures occurred when preparing the femoral canal or component placement. Intraoperative fractures that occur during hip arthroplasty can lead to worse outcomes, prolonged recovery, and increased risk of future revision surgeries.[3–5] With the projected increase of both primary and revision THA, we

---

Department of Orthopedic Surgery, NYU Langone Health, 301 East 17th Street, 15th Floor Suite 1518, New York, NY 10003, USA
* Corresponding author.
E-mail address: Ran.Schwarzkopf@nyulangone.org

Orthop Clin N Am 55 (2024) 19–26
https://doi.org/10.1016/j.ocl.2023.05.010

can expect to continue witnessing these intraoperative complications.[6,7]

The treatment of intraoperative trochanteric fractures varies with options ranging from nonoperative management to reduction and fixation of the fracture using wires, cables, plates, or a combination of fixation strategies. Treatment modality can depend on fracture morphology and surgeon preference. Greater trochanteric fractures tend to displace owing to the strong force of the attached abductor muscles.[8] Previous literature has shown that nonoperative management is an option for certain fracture morphologies.[9,10] However, for patients with displaced fractures or those who are more active, reduction and fixation of the fracture is often necessary. The surgical options for the treatment of intraoperative trochanteric fractures include internal fixation with cerclage wiring, cabling, screws, or plating techniques.[11,12]

Intraoperative trochanteric fractures during primary and revision THA can be serious complications that can occur during any part of the procedure. These complications can lead to worse outcomes and longer hospital stays. Therefore, it is essential to accurately identify and manage these fractures when seen in the operating room. In this article, the authors review intraoperative management, treatment strategies, and postoperative protocol for patients who have intraoperative trochanteric fractures.

PATIENT EVALUATION

Although intraoperative trochanteric fractures most often occur during the preparation of the femoral canal or component placement, patients can be at risk of fracture during any part of the procedure. Therefore, surgeons should have a high index of suspicion particularly when performing uncemented revision THA. Adequate exposure and visualization of the hip before dislocation and during femoral canal preparation can allow for improved identification of trochanteric fractures. Depending on the morphology of the fracture, a surgeon may feel a change in resistance when broaching or inserting the femoral stem.[13] This is particularly evident with trochanteric fractures that extend distally to the metaphysis. In the setting of revision THA, trochanteric fractures can also arise during the removal of well-fixed femoral components.[14] The use of changes in acoustic vibrations when broaching and placing the stem can also alert the surgeon of possible periprosthetic fractures intraoperatively.[15]

Once an intraoperative trochanteric fracture is identified, the surgeon must evaluate the size, location, extension, and displacement of the fragment. These characteristics can influence the type of treatment chosen. In addition, a patient's preoperative activity level can also play a role in the treatment of these fractures. To aid in the evaluation of the morphology of the fracture, surgeons may use radiographic imaging. Imaging can assist in quantifying the amount of fracture extension that may not be seen with direct visualization, although nondisplaced fractures may be better appreciated on imaging.[16] However, imaging may be limited based on tables designed with central posts that can block access to mobile imaging units, such as C-arm.[17] Regardless of the treatment method used, the femoral component stability must be evaluated before the completion of the procedure.

The senior author prefers direct visualization of the trochanteric fracture and will carefully retract soft tissues and expose the femur distally to identify the distal extent of the fracture. If necessary, the incision can also be extended distally to aid in visualization. If the fracture occurs during canal broaching and has distal extension, the broach is removed, and distal fixation, typically in the form of cables or wires, is applied to avoid extension of the fracture. Alternatively, when a trochanteric fracture occurs during final implant placement, the senior author will remove the implant and assess fracture morphology. Distal fixation typically in the form of cables or wires will be applied to prophylactically prevent fracture propagation before implanting the femoral component.

TREATMENT
Conservative Management
Many of the recommendations about conservative management come from literature assessing postoperative periprosthetic trochanteric fractures. In the setting of small, minimally displaced trochanteric fractures, conservative management may be an option for a small group of patients. This treatment may be an option for patients with low preoperative physical demand. Nonsurgical management should be reserved for truly minimally displaced trochanteric fractures because greater than 2 cm of displacement can significantly affect the biomechanics of the abductor complex (Fig. 1).[18] Patients should be educated about postoperative activity precautions, which include partial weight-bearing and avoiding abduction to prevent displacement of the fracture fragment.[19] Given these restrictions, patients may be slower to progress and require additional resources for safe discharge and rehabilitation.

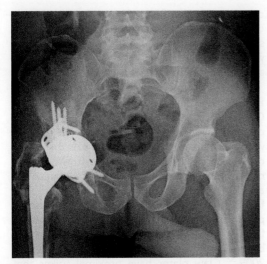

Fig. 1. Anteroposterior radiograph of a pelvis demonstrating a minimally displaced trochanter fracture sustained intraoperatively treated conservatively.

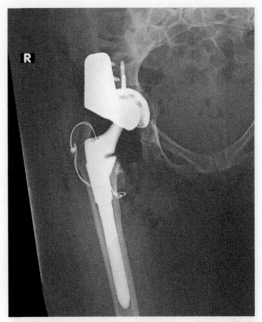

Fig. 2. Anteroposterior radiograph of the right hip with isolated greater trochanter fracture secured with wire fixation in a figure-of-eight formation.

Wire and Cable Fixation

Wires and cables for greater trochanter fractures have long been used for fracture fixation. These fixation strategies offer surgeons a method of applying compression to the fracture site.[20] In addition, wires and cables can be used in the setting of isolated trochanteric fractures with well-fixed femoral stems. Fracture patterns amenable to reduction and compression are amenable to this form of fixation. Reduction clamps can be used to achieve initial reduction of the fracture fragment. Once a reduction is achieved, wiring can be used to achieve adequate compression across the fracture site, such as the Charnley wiring technique.[21] This technique uses multiple wires in more than one plane producing a secure, compressive construct.

If using cables, 2 cables can be passed over the greater trochanter and both above and below the lesser trochanter. The cables are then progressively tensioned to achieve adequate compression. The cables can alternatively be secured in a figure-of-eight formation (Fig. 2). In the setting of trochanteric fractures with distal extension, cerclage cables can be applied circumferentially around the distal extension of the fracture to mitigate the risk of fracture propagation (Fig. 3). When used by the senior author for the prevention of fracture propagation, the broach or implant is typically removed before placement of the implant to ensure adequate reduction and stabilization of the fracture. Both these fixation strategies have some disadvantages. Wires are at risk of breakage and migration particularly with any

kinking and can be difficult to adequately tighten.[22,23] Cable fixation has been demonstrated to have low nonunion rates compared with other fixation methods and provides better compression but is also at risk of breaking and migrating.[24,25]

Cable Grip Fixation

Cable grip fixation offers a solution for many morphologies of greater trochanteric fractures in both the primary and the revision settings. The addition of these cable grips over the trochanteric fractures allows their claw design to secure the fracture fragment. Once the fracture is reduced, the cables can be sequentially tightened to improve the rigidity and fixation of the construct.[26] In addition to fracture fixation, cable grip systems allow for the fixation of allograft to aid in fracture healing.[27] Similar to cerclage cable fixation, this method also has a higher risk of hardware breakage and migration (Fig. 4).[24] However, relative to cable fixation alone, cable grip fixation is able to withstand a maximum load 1.5 times greater than that of cables alone.[28] When using a cable grip fixation method, surgeons should be cautious and use good operative techniques to avoid early failure. An intact medial cortex distal to the lesser trochanter should be present when using this fixation method, and if there is proximal medial bone loss, care must be taken to avoid direct

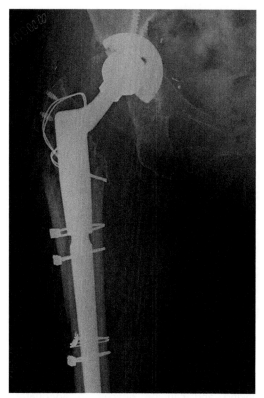

Fig. 3. Anteroposterior radiograph of the right hip with greater trochanter fracture with distal extension secured with greater trochanter fixation with wire in a figure-of-eight formation and distal cerclage cables.

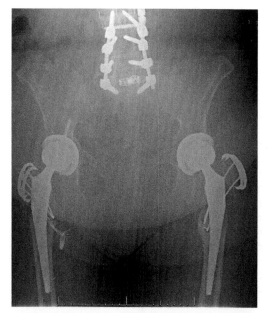

Fig. 4. Anteroposterior radiograph of a pelvis demonstrating bilateral hardware failure of cable grip fixation.

contact with the femoral stem to avoid early cable failure.[20] Using larger cable diameters significantly reduces the risk of early failure with 2.0-mm cables having half the rate of failure as 1.6-mm cables.[29]

Plate Fixation

Greater trochanteric fractures with comminution or severe osteolysis may not be amenable to wire or cable fixation strategies. For these and other complicated trochanteric fractures, plating can be used to adequately reduce and maintain a reduction. The most commonly described plate for trochanteric fixation in the literature is the claw plate design.[30–32] The use of locking plates for the fixation of greater trochanter fractures has also been used with one of the first reported cases in 2009.[33] Claw plates have proximal spikes that allow surgeons to capture the greater trochanter fragment and maintain reduction (Fig. 5). Locking plates use multiple locking screws in multiple planes to secure the greater trochanter fragment to the plate. When comparing plate fixation and cable fixation, a biomechanical study found that plating was more biomechanically stable than cable fixation.[34]

Although claw plates have been widely used, there has been some debate on the efficacy of this fixation method. Zarin and colleagues [32] performed a retrospective review of 31 patients using a claw plate for reattachment of the greater trochanter and concluded that they offered an effective method to reconstruct the greater trochanter in the setting of nonunion and periprosthetic fracture. A 10-year follow-up study looking at primary and revision THA found that patients continued to show clinical benefits after reduction using a claw plate.[30] However, some studies have shown that plating may have high rates of nonunion or migration of the fracture fragment.[24,35]

POSTOPERATIVE MANAGEMENT

Following successful reduction and fixation of an intraoperative trochanteric fracture, a patient's activity level must be modified to prevent displacement of the fracture. Previous literature has recommended that patients with these types of fracture have limited weight-bearing for several weeks and then transition to full weight-bearing by 6 weeks.[36–38] Tetreault and McGrory[36] recommended that patients avoid active abduction for 6 weeks postoperatively owing to the risk of fragment displacement.

The senior author of this article similarly maintains patients on partial weight-bearing for

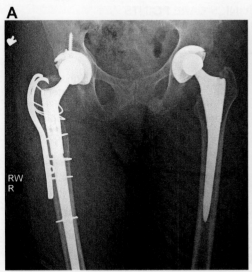

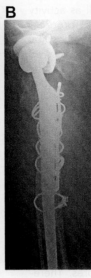

Fig. 5. (A) Anteroposterior and (B) lateral radiographs demonstrating claw plate and cerclage cable fixation of a trochanteric fracture during a revision THA.

6 weeks postoperatively with the assistance of a walker and advises against active abduction. Patients are seen in clinic, and images in the form of anteroposterior and lateral hip radiographs are taken at 6 weeks and 3 months. The senior author uses these radiographs for surveillance of the fracture to assess complications and fracture healing. After 6 weeks and with maintained reduction on hip radiographs, patients are permitted to fully weight-bear and actively abduct the operative extremity. Similar to previous studies, union is considered when there is evidence of bone bridging on hip radiographs and there is minimal to no discomfort with weight-bearing.[36,39]

OUTCOMES AND COMPLICATIONS

There has been little consensus on the reported outcomes of intraoperative trochanteric fractures during primary and revision THA. Studies have reported on the successful treatment of greater trochanteric fractures with high rates of union and improved patient-reported outcomes.[32,36] Schafer and colleagues[40] demonstrated a union

rate of 76.3% after greater trochanteric fracture fixation in primary and revision THA. This study also found that improved anatomic positioning of the cable plate and increasing the number of cables used may increase the rate of successful fixation. Another study examined 15 intraoperative greater trochanter fractures treated with fixation and demonstrated successful union in all patients with some patients experiencing only a slight limp.[41] Similarly, patients who sustained intraoperative fractures during revision THA had similar Western Ontario and McMaster Universities Osteoarthritis Index, Oxford-12, and Short Form-36 scores when compared with patients who did not have intraoperative fractures during revision THA.[42]

Although several studies have demonstrated success in the treatment of intraoperative trochanteric fractures, several studies have highlighted the poor outcomes and complications that can arise from trochanteric fractures and the method of fixation. Postoperative pain and abductor weakness can often lead to poor outcomes after fracture fixation, particularly when using plate fixation methods.[24,43] With increased

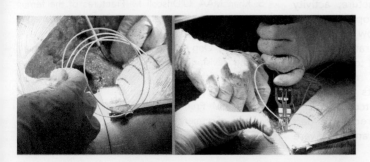

Fig. 6. Intraoperative images of a nylon cable used for fixation in a revision THA in the setting of a periprosthetic joint infection.

pain and abductor weakness as well as activity restrictions, patients may be slow to progress with therapy and have extended hospital stays.[44] Neitzke and colleagues[31] demonstrated that 12 of 22 patients with greater trochanteric periprosthetic fractures treated with operative repair had complications, with 7 patients requiring reoperation.

Wire and cable fixation methods are at risk of breakage leading to fracture displacement and nonunion.[24] Moreover, third-body wear owing to breakage of cables or wires can lead to early failure of the THA owing to polyethylene wear and loosening in the setting of osteolysis.[45,46] This complication may lead to increased reoperation rates. Although hardware failure can occur, Kim and colleagues[47] demonstrated that patients who have a nonunion after fixation can still have improvement in Harris hip scores. Therefore, patients with hardware failure should be closely monitored for evidence of worsening pain or radiographic evidence of hip implant complications owing to metal debris.

SUMMARY

Intraoperative trochanteric fractures during primary and revision THA can occur during any part of the procedure and can lead to worse patient outcomes. It is important that these fractures are accurately identified during the procedure to allow the surgeon to choose the appropriate treatment option. Surgeons should weigh patient-specific factors, such as preoperative activity level and bone density as well as fracture morphology, when choosing fixation strategies. In addition to the previously mentioned treatment options, newer technologies have been introduced to assist in fracture fixation particularly in the revision setting. These include modular THA stems with trochanteric plates that can be bolted to the implant directly and nonmetallic cables, such as nylon or ultra-high-molecular-weight polyethylene fiber cables, which can be useful in periprosthetic joint infection cases (Fig. 6).[48–50] After treatment of a trochanteric fracture, activity levels should be modified postoperatively to limit active abduction and allow for partial weight-bearing through the operative extremity. Patients should be counseled to ensure understanding of postoperative rehabilitation protocols and the adverse effects trochanteric fractures can have on patient outcomes. Close follow-up with radiographs is recommended to assess fracture displacement and hardware complications.

CLINICS CARE POINTS

- Surgeons should have a high level of suspicion for intraoperative trochanteric fractures particularly in the setting of uncemented revision total hip arthroplasty.
- There is little consensus on the outcomes of patients who have intraoperative trochanteric fractures during total hip arthroplasty, and patients should be informed of the possibility of poorer clinical outcomes.
- Hardware failure is a major complication of all fixation strategies and should be closely surveilled with clinical follow-up and radiographs.

DECLARATION OF CONFLICTING INTERESTS

A. Habibi. has nothing to disclose. R. Schwarzkopf. reports IP royalties from Smith & Nephew, being a paid consultant for Smith & Nephew and Intellijoint, having stock options from Intellijoint and Gauss Surgical, and receiving research support from Smith & Nephew, United States.

REFERENCES

1. Berry DJ. EPIDEMIOLOGY: Hip and Knee. Orthop Clin N Am 1999;30(2):183–90.
2. Abdel MP, Watts CD, Houdek MT, et al. Epidemiology of periprosthetic fracture of the femur in 32 644 primary total hip arthroplasties: a 40-year experience. Bone Joint Lett J 2016;98-B(4):461–7.
3. Sheth NP, Brown NM, Moric M, et al. Operative Treatment of Early Peri-Prosthetic Femur Fractures Following Primary Total Hip Arthroplasty. J Arthroplasty 2013;28(2):286–91.
4. Thillemann TM, Pedersen AB, Johnsen SP, et al. Inferior outcome after intraoperative femoral fracture in total hip arthroplasty. New Pub: Medical Journals Sweden. Acta Orthop 2009;79(3):327–34.
5. Khan MAA, O'Driscoll M. Fractures of the femur during total hip replacement and their management. J Bone Joint Surg Br 1977;59(1):36–41.
6. Kurtz S, Ong K, Lau E, et al. Projections of primary and revision hip and knee arthroplasty in the United States from 2005 to 2030. J Bone Joint Surg 2007;89(4):780–5.
7. Sloan M, Premkumar A, Sheth NP. Projected volume of primary total joint arthroplasty in the U.S., 2014 to 2030. Journal of Bone and Joint Surgery - American 2018;100(17):1455–60.

8. Pagnano M. Intra-operative fractures during THA: see it before it sees you. Orthopaedic Proceedings. Published February 21, 2018. Available at: https://online.boneandjoint.org.uk/doi/abs/10.1302/1358-992x.98bsupp_22.ccjr2015-019. Accessed January 23, 2023.

9. Hartford JM, Graw BP, Knowles SB, et al. Isolated Greater Trochanteric Fracture and the Direct Anterior Approach Using a Fracture Table. J Arthroplasty 2018;33(7):S253–8.

10. Pritchett JW. Fracture of the greater trochanter after hip replacement. Clin Orthop Relat Res 2001; 390(390):221–6.

11. Sun D, Park BS, Jang GI, et al. The Fixation Method according to the Fracture Type of the Greater Trochanter in Unstable Intertrochanteric Fractures Undergoing Arthroplasty. Hip Pelvis 2017;29(1):62.

12. Huang G, Zhang M, Qu Z, et al. Fixation options for reconstruction of the greater trochanter in unstable intertrochanteric fracture with arthroplasty. Medicine 2021;100(26):E26395.

13. Siddiqi A, Springer BD, Chen AF, et al. Diagnosis and Management of Intraoperative Fractures in Primary Total Hip Arthroplasty. J Am Acad Orthop Surg 2021;29(10):e497–512.

14. Abdel MP, Wyles CC, Viste A, et al. Extended Trochanteric Osteotomy in Revision Total Hip Arthroplasty: Contemporary Outcomes of 612 Hips. J Bone Joint Surg 2021;103(2):162–73.

15. Wei JCJ, Crezee WHA, Jongeneel H, et al. Using Acoustic Vibrations as a Method for Implant Insertion Assessment in Total Hip Arthroplasty. Sensors 2022;22(4):1609.

16. Davidson D, Pike J, Garbuz D, et al. Intraoperative periprosthetic fractures during total hip arthroplasty: Evaluation and management. J Bone Joint Surg 2008;90(9):2000–12.

17. Habibi AA, Bi AS, Owusu-Sarpong S, et al. History, indications, and advantages of orthopaedic operating room tables: a review. Eur J Orthop Surg Traumatol 2022;32(6):1207–13.

18. Marsland D, Mears SC. A Review of Periprosthetic Femoral Fractures Associated With Total Hip Arthroplasty. Geriatr Orthop Surg Rehabil 2011. https://doi.org/10.1177/2151458512462870.

19. Ricci WM, Borrelli J. Operative management of periprosthetic femur fractures in the elderly using biological fracture reduction and fixation techniques. Injury 2007;38(Suppl 3):53–8.

20. Jarit GJ, Sathappan SS, Panchal A, et al. Fixation systems of greater trochanteric osteotomies: biomechanical and clinical outcomes. J Am Acad Orthop Surg 2007;15(10):614–24.

21. Charnley J, Ferreiraade S. TRANSPLANTATION OF THE GREATER TROCHANTER IN ARTHROPLASTY OF THE HIP. J Bone Joint Surg Br 1964;46:191–7.

22. Amstutz HC, Mai LL, Schmidt I. Results of interlocking wire trochanteric reattachment and technique refinements to prevent complications following total hip arthroplasty. Clin Orthop Relat Res 1984; 183(183):82–9.

23. Boardman KP, Bocco F, Charnley J. An evaluation of a method of trochanteric fixation using three wires in the Charnley low friction arthroplasty. Clin Orthop Relat Res 1978;132(132):31–8.

24. Mei XY, Gong YJ, Safir OA, et al. Fixation Options Following Greater Trochanteric Osteotomies and Fractures in Total Hip Arthroplasty: A Systematic Review. JBJS Rev 2018;6(6):e4.

25. Ritter MA, Eizember LE, Keating EM, et al. Trochanteric fixation by cable grip in hip replacement. J Bone Joint Surg Br 1991;73(4):580–1.

26. Barrack RL, Butler RA. Current status of trochanteric reattachment in complex total hip arthroplasty. Clin Orthop Relat Res 2005;441:237–42.

27. Dall DM. A Biomechanical and Clinical Review: The Dall-Miles Cable System. Treatment of Osteoarthritic Change in the Hip 2007;239–50. https://doi.org/10.1007/978-4-431-38200-3_24.

28. Hersh CK, Williams RP, Trick LW, et al. Comparison of the mechanical performance of trochanteric fixation devices. Clin Orthop Relat Res 1996;329(329):317–25.

29. Dall DM, Miles AW. Re-attachment of the greater trochanter. The use of the trochanter cable-grip system. J Bone Joint Surg Br 1983;65(1):55–9.

30. Tang J, Wu T, Shao H, et al. Greater trochanter fixed with a claw plate and cable system in complex primary and revision total hip arthroplasty: long-term f-up. Int Orthop 2022;46(11):2553–60.

31. Neitzke C, Davis E, Puri S, et al. Contemporary Use of Trochanteric Plates in Periprosthetic Femur Fractures: A Displaced Trochanter Will Not Be Tamed. J Arthroplasty 2023;38(1):158–64.

32. Zarin JS, Zurakowski D, Burke DW. Claw plate fixation of the greater trochanter in revision total hip arthroplasty. J Arthroplasty 2009;24(2):272–80.

33. McGrory BJ, Lucas R. The use of locking plates for greater trochanteric fixation. Orthopedics 2009; 32(12):917.

34. Sariyilmaz K, Korkmaz M, Özkunt O, et al. Comparison of fixation techniques in Vancouver type AG periprosthetic femoral fracture: a biomechanical study. Acta Orthop Traumatol Turc 2016;50(3):373–8.

35. Stewart AD, Abdelbary H, Beaulé PE. Trochanteric Fixation With a Third-Generation Cable-Plate System: An Independent Experience. J Arthroplasty 2017;32(9):2864–8.e1.

36. Tetreault AK, McGrory BJ. Use of locking plates for fixation of the greater trochanter in patients with hip replacement. Arthroplast Today 2016;2(4):187–92.

37. Hsieh PH, Chang YH, Lee PC, et al. Periprosthetic fractures of the greater trochanter through osteolytic cysts with uncemented MicroStructured Omnifit prosthesis: retrospective analyses pf 23 fractures in 887 hips after 5-14 years. Acta Orthop 2005;76(4):538–43.

38. Brozovich A, Lionberger DR. Periprosthetic Fracture of Greater Trochanter in Total Hip Replacement Stemming from Pin Site Placement in Navigation-Assisted Surgery. Case Rep Orthop 2019;2019:1–6.

39. Old AB, McGrory BJ, White RR, et al. Fixation of Vancouver B1 peri-prosthetic fractures by broad metal plates without the application of strut allografts. J Bone Joint Surg Br 2006;88(11):1425–9.

40. Schafer P, Sullivan TC, Lambert B, et al. Greater Trochanteric Fixation Using Cable Plate Devices in Complex Primary and Revision Total Hip Arthroplasty. Arthroplast Today 2023;20:101103.

41. Hendel D, Yasin M, Garti A, et al. Fracture of the greater trochanter during hip replacement. Clin Orthop Relat Res 2009;73(3):295–7.

42. Meek RMD, Garbuz DS, Masri BA, et al. Intraoperative fracture of the femur in revision total hip arthroplasty with a diaphyseal fitting stem. J Bone Joint Surg Am 2004;86(3):480–5.

43. Peretz JI, Chuang MJ, Cerynik DL, et al. Treatment of Symptomatic Greater Trochanteric Fracture After Total Hip Arthroplasty. J Arthroplasty 2009;24(5):825.e1–4.

44. Marino D v., Mesko DR. Periprosthetic Proximal Femur Fractures. StatPearls. Published online September 25, 2022. Available at: https://www.ncbi.nlm.nih.gov/books/NBK557559/. Accessed January 31, 2023.

45. Kelley SS, Johnston RC. Debris From Cobalt-Chrome Cable May Cause Acetabular Loosening. Clin Orthop Relat Res 1992;285:140–6.

46. Altenburg AJ, Callaghan JJ, Yehyawi TM, et al. Cemented Total Hip Replacement Cable Debris and Acetabular Construct Durability. J Bone Joint Surg Am 2009;91(7):1664.

47. Kim IS, Pansey N, Kansay RK, et al. Greater Trochanteric Reattachment Using the Third-Generation Cable Plate System in Revision Total Hip Arthroplasty. J Arthroplasty 2017;32(6):1965–9.

48. Hedlundh U, Karlsson L. Combining a hip arthroplasty stem with trochanteric reattachment bolt and a polyaxial locking plate in the treatment of a periprosthetic fracture below a well-integrated implant. Arthroplast Today 2016;2(4):141–5.

49. Oe K, Iida H, Kobayashi F, et al. Reattachment of an osteotomized greater trochanter in total hip arthroplasty using an ultra-high molecular weight polyethylene fiber cable. J Orthop Sci 2018;23(6):992–9.

50. Speranza A, Massafra C, Pecchia S, et al. Metallic versus non-metallic cerclage cables system in periprosthetic hip fracture treatment: single-institution experience at a minimum 1-year follow-up. J Clin Med 2022;11(6):1608.

Intraoperative Challenges of the Kinematic Knee

Nicholas M. Brown, MD[a],*, Nithya Lingampalli, MD[a], Michael D. Hellman, MD[b],1

KEYWORDS

- Total knee replacement • Arthroplasty • Kinematic knee

KEY POINTS

- A kinematic knee replacement restores the unique pre-disease alignment and three dimensional rotational axes of a patient's pre-arthritic knee.
- The technique calls for calipering the resected fragments to replace with combined thickness of cartilage, bone, and saw kerf with the femoral component thickness.
- The technique is simple but requires a comprehensive understanding of the theory behind it to correctly make intraoperative adjustments to restore a more natural joint.

INTRODUCTION

A kinematic knee replacement restores the unique pre-disease alignment and rotational axes of a patient's knee.[1] This is in contrast to a mechanically aligned total knee arthroplasty (TKA) that aims for a neutral hip–knee–ankle alignment and a joint line perpendicular to the mechanical axes of each bone.[2,3] A kinematic knee replacement rests on the assumption that a diseased femur can be reproducibly resurfaced to its pre-diseased state by assuming that native cartilage is 2 mm thick. Therefore, the total amount of cartilage wear in addition to the bone and cartilage cut away, should equal the thickness of the implant replacing the resections.[4] Although there are many variations of this technique (inverse kinematic, functional alignment, restricted kinematic, anatomic, and so forth), the specific unrestricted kinematic alignment technique, we are focusing on, is described in the following references.[1,5–9] Although this is a simple, easily adoptable technique, there are, of course, many preoperative and intraoperative challenges that may arise.

PREOPERATIVE CHALLENGES

One of the first challenges is determining which patients are appropriate candidates for this technique. The answer is that 90% or more of patients will be within 3 degrees of neutral on their hip–knee–ankle alignment, and can be effectively treated using this method.[10–12] The choice to use this technique for the rare cases of severe valgus disease, post-traumatic deformity, hyperlaxity, and childhood knee disease can be left up to the individual surgeon's discretion and comfort as many times the case can be performed utilizing both kinematic and traditional mechanical methods.[13]

The second typically encountered preoperative challenge is the belief that additional imaging is needed beyond the standard 4 radiographic views of the knee obtained in the clinic. Many surgeons have a misconception that adopting this technique will require additional advanced imaging or long leg alignment films to measure the angles of the planned cuts in the coronal plane. However, this is unnecessary for a variety of reasons: one, there is inherent error in the measurements templated from

---

a Loyola University Medical Center, 2160 South 1st Avenue #3328, Maywood, IL 60153, USA; b Lees Summit, MO, USA

1 Present address: 2160 South 1st Avenue #3328, Maywood, IL 60153

* Corresponding author.

E-mail address: nmb2116@gmail.com

Orthop Clin N Am 55 (2024) 27–32
https://doi.org/10.1016/j.ocl.2023.07.001

imaging due to variation in rotation, angulation, bone loss, and human error. Rather than obtaining measurements and attempting to translate these to cut angles, the cut guides are physically placed on fully visualized bony and cartilaginous surfaces intraoperatively to increase the probability of making accurate cuts. The exact values of the angles are in and of themselves unimportant, but rather restoring the native geometry, alignment, and balance of the patient's knee is paramount. This can be easily and reproducibly performed with standard instruments and radiographs.

Intraoperative Challenges
Distal Femoral Cut
The first challenge encountered with making the distal femoral cut is to appropriately place the intramedullary rod without significant flexion or extension in relation to the axis of the knee. Options include using a shorter or more flexible guide rod or restricting the depth of insertion into the canal. It is also crucial to be cognizant of creating a starting hole and entering the canal approximately 5 to 10 mm above the notch. Entering the femoral canal more anterior or posterior to this point may cause the component to be placed in flexion or extension, which may affect range of motion, patellar tracking, and overall satisfaction.

The next challenge is placing the distal femoral guide flat on the distal femur and accurately accounting for cartilage loss on the worn side of the femur. Although some systems are designed with special cutting guides or shims to account for the cartilage thickness, any object with approximately 2 mm of thickness can function effectively as a spacer. Before placing the femoral guide, it is important to remove any osteophytes creating an uneven surface that prevents the guide from sitting flush on the bone. If the cartilage is partially worn on either the "worn" or "unworn" sides of the femur, options are to remove the residual cartilage with a curette or adjust for the residual thickness when making the cut. For example, if the cartilage is worn on both medial and lateral condyles, the surgeon would set the distal femoral cut guide to remove 2 mm less than normal to account for the bilateral wear.

A final challenge arises when the distal femoral cutting guide limits the valgus alignment such that the lateral distal femoral condyle is under-resected. Many surgeons choose to use a system that allows for a full range of distal femoral cutting angles to avoid this potential problem. However, if using a system that does not allow cutting beyond a certain angle, this can be dealt with by pinning the guide medially and pivoting on the pin. Alternatively, if the distal femoral condyle is under-resected, the posterior lateral condyle can be concurrently under-resected by the same amount to avoid a flexion–extension mismatch when balancing the knee. This would be considered more of a restricted kinematic technique.

After you complete your distal femoral cut, it is necessary to verify the cut with a caliper. A correct cut should be approximately 1 mm less than your intended cut due to the kerf of the blade accounting for 1 mm. If you cut too little, it is important to pass the saw again either through the guide or free hand to have a correctly resected segment. If your cut is too much, you can restore the surface of the distal femur by placing a shim, such as a 1 mm washer, on the 4-in-1 cut block so that your chamfer cuts correct the over-resection. If you resected 3 mm too much, we recommend considering placing multiple short (10–14 mm) small frag screws into the surface of the over-resected distal femur. Small frag screw heads are 3 mm and washers are 1 mm. These inexpensive "augments" help restore the correct position of the distal femur and act as rebar for the cement.

Anterior, Posterior, and Chamfer Cuts
The most significant challenge encountered with this step is when determining whether there is cartilage on the posterior femur that must then be accounted for by posterior shims on the femoral sizing guide. From our experience with unicompartmental knee arthroplasty, a valgus knee often is a "disease of flexion," with the true extent of cartilage wear visualized best on weight-bearing flexion films.[14] Therefore, with valgus knees, the surgeon must often account for lost cartilage or even bone in severe cases. However, there is often cartilage on the medial posterior condyle unless the ACL has been incompetent for a prolonged period of time, if there is varus subluxation, or if there is a severe disease. In either case, the authors find the amount of residual cartilage present posteriorly is best assessed with a scalpel or measuring probe with the knee in maximal flexion.

Tibial Cut
There are 3 challenges that need to be overcome before cutting the tibia: axially rotating the anterior–posterior axis of the tibial cut plane to parallel the flexion–extension plane of the native knee, sagittally rotating the tibial cut plane to parallel the slope of the native tibia,

and coronally rotating the tibial cut plane to parallel the native proximal varus angle. Traditional landmarks such as the medial one-third of the tibial tubercle do not reliably assist the surgeon to find the correct axial rotation for the tibial cut plane.[15] The correct axial rotation can be found by referencing the anterior–posterior axis of the lateral tibial plateau.[16] When the tibia is exposed through anterior subluxation, an ellipse can be drawn around the lateral tibial plateau. The center of this ellipse best matches the flexion–extension axis of the native knee. Therefore, the axial rotation of the tibial cut plane should parallel this reference line. Finding the native tibial slope plane can be difficult due to significant wear of the tibial articular surface, osteophytes, and differences in slope between the medial and lateral tibial condyles.[17–20] Determination of tibial slope is best achieved by referencing the medial tibial spine. One can place a k-wire along the base of the medial tibial spine, which gives you a reference line to parallel, alternatively one can use the stylus and run it anterior to posterior along the base of the medial tibial spine. If the stylus evenly touches the tibia and does not dig in posteriorly or lift off posterior, your slope is likely correct. You can also place an angel wing inside the tibial cut guide and have the finger run along the medial border of the tibia. The lateral radiograph can be used as a reference; however, variations in leg rotation, radiographic angulation, and tibial bone loss can confound the accuracy of the measured tibial slope. Rather than aiming for a particular number, an accurate slope is when the knee is balanced in full extension, and the posterior cruciate ligament (PCL) is appropriately tensioned in flexion. It is important to be judicious when re-creating slope, as the excessive slope is a potential cause of tibial failure and may be restricted even in cases when an "unrestricted kinematic knee" is being performed.[21,22] However, the acceptable limit of slope is controversial and more study is needed to understand a clinically validated limit in a kinematic knee. The accuracy of the slope cut can be assessed by verifying the symmetry of the anterior and posterior tibial bone on the cut piece.

The final challenge is to properly recreate the varus–valgus angle of the tibia. For the limitations previously mentioned, radiographs provide only a rough approximation. In an ACL-competent varus knee, the wear pattern is commonly anteromedial and there is usually some cartilage remaining posteriorly.[23–25] However, in cases of severe wear or bone loss, the angle is more challenging to set. There is often cartilage remaining along the tibial spines, even in cases of severe wear, and it may be a helpful, consistent landmark. Other surgeons elect to measure a 7 mm cut located exactly at the tidemark of tibial cartilage wear. This technique is based on the assumption that while the tibia, unlike the femur, may have bone loss in areas where measurements are obtained, there is unlikely to be bone loss right at the tidemark.

Flexion–Extension Imbalance. Occasionally, a patient will have physiologic hyperextension that causes a perceived imbalance. Leaving a patient in their slight native hyperextension is acceptable and not known to cause problems. However, if the hyperextension is due to the over-resection of the distal femur, the femoral component can be distalized on the cement with an extra cement buffer. Another scenario that can be encountered is when the knee is loose in extension, or equivalently tight in flexion, due to a tight PCL. The first step is to ensure that there are no osteophytes impinging on the PCL. If the PCL is free of impinging structures, the next step is to reassess your tibial cut and ensure that the correct slope was cut. If you note less resection of the posterior tibia than the anterior tibia, you should cut an additional slope. Once the native tibial slope has been reached, the PCL can be partially resected until the balance is restored. Partial resection can occur at the femoral side. Place the knee at 90 degrees and feather the PCL at the medial femoral notch while applying a force-directed posterior on the tibia. Once you feel the femur "roll forward," you can stop the resection. If the PCL is partially resected, consideration should be given to using a medial pivot or ultra-congruent polyethylene insert that does not rely on PCL integrity for flexion stability. However, it should be noted that it is rare that the PCL is inherently "tight," as it is typically the bone cuts altering the native anatomy that has led to its tightness.

A more commonly encountered scenario is a knee tighter in extension due to a residual flexion contracture. It is important to resist the urge to resect additional distal femur unless the contracture is pathologic and greater than 25 to 30 degrees. This is because the majority of flexion contractures are due to osteophytes tensioning soft tissue or a contracted posterior capsule and not a result of distal femoral overgrowth.[26–29] With appropriate cuts, osteophyte resection, and occasional posterior capsular release, the vast majority of flexion contractures will resolve.

Varus–Valgus Imbalance. The knee is often equally balanced in extension and has a slightly increased lateral laxity in flexion. A spacer block should be used to assess your balance after all cuts have been completed. First, in 90 degrees of flexion, the spacer block should feel like it pivots around the medial side. Second, in full extension, the spacer block should show no varus or valgus laxity. And finally, at about 30 degrees of flexion, there should be 3 to 4 mm of laxity on the lateral side with varus and valgus pressure. If the knee is imbalanced and the native femoral anatomy has been restored, balance is obtained by cutting more varus or valgus alignment into the tibia. Some manufacturers provide recut guides in their sets for this purpose. However, if these are unavailable, a recut can be performed by dropping the block to the lower pin holes, rotating around the appropriate fixation pin, and re-pinning the guide into the new position with increased varus or valgus angulation. The challenge at this step is to understand whether the balance is due to malrestoration of the native tibial anatomy or due to ligaments that have stretched. In most cases, ligaments are not altered from their native length and tension and balance are restored by adjusting the tibial cuts. However, there are cases of severe deformity or pathologic anatomy where ligaments have stretched. In these instances, compromises should be made with extra constraint or ligamentous release. Surgeons interested in this technique are often hesitant to adopt it, citing the extreme position the tibial component would require to balance the knee in these cases. In reality, these situations are rare, and the goal is to restore native anatomy, not simply balance the knee through tibial cuts in all scenarios. Further, there are a multitude of studies demonstrating excellent mid-term survivorship in patients with no restrictions in their coronal tibial alignment.[30–32]

Medial–Lateral Imbalance Flexion Versus Extension

The traditional goal of TKA, particularly one performed with a gap-balanced technique, is to have equal balance medially and laterally that is maintained throughout flexion and extension. This is the "feel" of the knee that many surgeons are trained and comfortable with, hence, deviating from this can be an intraoperative challenge. However, it is well understood and documented that the native knee is most taut in extension and slightly looser through flexion, more so laterally than medially in a variable manner.[33,34] Nowakowski and

colleagues[35] published a gap of approximately 6.8 ± 1.0 mm medially and 9.2 ± 1.1 mm laterally. Additionally, this variable loosening in flexion is appreciated by any surgeon who performs knee arthroscopy—obtaining access to the lateral compartment is easy with the knee in flexion (figure of 4 position), while the medial compartment remains difficult to access when the knee is flexed. As a result of restoring the native knee anatomy and alignment, the length–tension relationships of the soft tissues are also reestablished, which will lead to this pattern of "native imbalance."

However, a situation can arise when performing this technique with conventional instrumentation where the native distal femoral valgus is beyond the allowance of the instrumentation. This can lead to over-resection of the medial distal condyle and under-resection of the lateral distal condyle. However, if the flexion axis is set based on the posterior condyles, and native rotation is restored, the knee will be tighter medially in flexion than extension. This imbalance can be solved either by ensuring the distal femoral cut is correct by adjusting the distal femoral cutting guide manually or by under-resecting in flexion the same amount that was under-resected in extension. This decision is based on the surgeon's comfort with manually making adjustments beyond the limits of conventional instrumentation. If the surgeon is not comfortable with manual modifications of the resection, it is important to account for this decision when setting the initial femoral cuts in flexion.

Patellar Tracking

If the patella is tracking well before the knee replacement and the native anatomy is closely restored, the patella should theoretically continue to track appropriately after the knee replacement. However, there are some situations that may arise that create patellar maltracking. The first obvious scenario is when the patellar tracking is abnormal before the knee replacement, which may be due to wear and altered alignment. The patellar tracking may correct to normal after the pre-disease anatomy has been restored without any additional steps. However, in cases where the pre-disease anatomy is abnormal such as with trochlear dysplasia, traditional techniques such as patellar resurfacing, component medialization, tibial component external rotation, or lateral release may be warranted. The author believes that the femoral anatomy should be restored as patellar maltracking is often due to underresection of the distal lateral femoral condyle, which causes over-tensioning of the lateral tissues.

There are 2 other scenarios the surgeon should be aware of that may contribute to patellar maltracking. One is an over-flexed femoral component that can cause maltracking due to late engagement of the patella into the trochlear groove. The second is inherent to the prosthetic design, as current artificial knee components are designed with the trochlear groove aligned with the axis of the condyles. However, in native knee anatomy, the posterior condylar axis is, on average, 3 degrees internally rotated in relation to the trochlear groove.[36] Therefore, the surgeon is making a concession and either recreating the femoral condylar anatomy or trochlear anatomy. If the condylar anatomy is recreated, the prosthetic trochlear groove will typically be internally rotated. It has been previously demonstrated that femoral component internal rotation may not be more associated with patellar maltracking when compared with external rotation.[37,38] Nevertheless, this potential problem should be recognized and accounted for by the surgeon in cases that may require slightly altering femoral rotation to correct maltracking.

SUMMARY

A thorough understanding of the anatomy and biomechanical principles underlying the concept of a kinematic knee is crucial in restoring the pre-disease alignment of a knee. A comprehensive approach beginning with a critical analysis of a patient's preoperative radiographs and physical examination sets the groundwork of identifying potential intraoperative complications for that the surgeon can create a game plan. A systematic intraoperative technique that analyzes the patient's unique disease characteristics aids in decision-making for resections and soft-tissue balancing with the ultimate goal of restoring the patient's pre-disease rotational and alignment axes.

CLINICS CARE POINTS

- 90% or more of patients will be within 3 degrees of neutral on their hip–knee–ankle alignment and can be effectively treated using the described kinematic knee replacement technique.
- No additional advanced imaging or long-leg alignment films beyond the standard knee radiographs is required to measure the angles of the planned cuts.
- Restoring the native knee anatomy and alignment, the length–tension relationships of the soft tissues are also reestablished, which will then lead to this pattern of "native imbalance."

DISCLOSURE

The authors have nothing to disclose.

REFERENCES

1. Weber P, Gollwitzer H. Kinematic alignment in total knee arthroplasty. Operat Orthop Traumatol 2021; 33(6):525–37.
2. Dossett HG, Swartz GJ, Estrada NA, et al. Kinematically versus mechanically aligned total knee arthroplasty. Orthopedics 2012;35(2):e160–9.
3. Lee YS, Howell SM, Won YY, et al. Kinematic alignment is a possible alternative to mechanical alignment in total knee arthroplasty. Knee Surg Sports Traumatol Arthrosc 2017;25(11):3467–79.
4. Howell SM, Hull ML, Nedopil AJ, et al. Caliper-verified kinematically aligned total knee arthroplasty: rationale, targets, accuracy, balancing, implant survival, and outcomes. Instr Course Lect 2023;72:241–59.
5. Winnock de Grave P, Kellens J, Luyckx T, et al. Inverse kinematic alignment for total knee arthroplasty. Orthop Traumatol Surg Res OTSR 2022; 108(5):103305.
6. Vendittoli PA, Martinov S, Blakeney WG. Restricted kinematic alignment, the fundamentals, and clinical applications. Front Surg 2021;8:697020.
7. Rivière C, Iranpour F, Auvinet E, et al. Alignment options for total knee arthroplasty: a systematic review. Orthop Traumatol Surg Res OTSR 2017; 103(7):1047–56.
8. Howell SM, Hull ML, Mahfouz MR. Kinematic alignment in total knee arthroplasty. In: Scott N, editor. *Insall and scott surgery of the knee*. Philadelphia: Elsevier; 2012. p. 1255–68.
9. Howell SM, Kuznik K, Hull ML, et al. Results of an initial experience with custom-fit positioning total knee arthroplasty in a series of 48 patients. Orthopedics 2008;31(9):857–63.
10. Eckhoff DG, Bach JM, Spitzer VM, et al. Three-dimensional morphology and kinematics of the distal part of the femur viewed in virtual reality. Part II. J Bone Joint Surg Am 2003;85-A(Suppl 4): 97–104.
11. Cooke D, Scudamore A, Li J, et al. Axial lower-limb alignment: comparison of knee geometry in normal volunteers and osteoarthritis patients. Osteoarthritis Cartilage 1997;5(1):39–47.

12. Moreland JR, Bassett LW, Hanker GJ. Radiographic analysis of the axial alignment of the lower extremity. J Bone Joint Surg Am 1987;69(5):745–9.

13. McEwen P, Balendra G, Doma K. Medial and lateral gap laxity differential in computer-assisted kinematic total knee arthroplasty. Bone Jt J 2019;101-B(3):331–9.

14. Rueckl K, Runer A, Bechler U, et al. The posterior-anterior-flexed view is essential for the evaluation of valgus osteoarthritis. A prospective study on 134 valgus knees. BMC Musculoskelet Disord 2019;20(1):636.

15. Brar AS, Howell SM, Hull ML. What are the bias, imprecision, and limits of agreement for finding the flexion-extension plane of the knee with five tibial reference lines? Knee 2016;23(3):406–11.

16. Howell SM, Papadopoulos S, Kuznik KT, et al. Accurate alignment and high function after kinematically aligned TKA performed with generic instruments. Knee Surg Sports Traumatol Arthrosc 2013;21(10): 2271–80.

17. Calek AK, Hochreiter B, Hess S, et al. High inter- and intraindividual differences in medial and lateral posterior tibial slope are not reproduced accurately by conventional TKA alignment techniques. Knee Surg Sports Traumatol Arthrosc 2022;30(3):882–9.

18. Okamoto S, Mizu-uchi H, Okazaki K, et al. Effect of tibial posterior slope on knee kinematics, quadriceps force, and patellofemoral contact force after posterior-stabilized total knee arthroplasty. J Arthroplasty 2015;30(8):1439–43.

19. Chambers AW, Wood AR, Kosmopoulos V, et al. Effect of posterior tibial slope on flexion and anterior-posterior tibial translation in posterior cruciate-retaining total knee arthroplasty. J Arthroplasty 2016;31(1):103–6.

20. Kang KT, Kwon SK, Son J, et al. Effects of posterior condylar offset and posterior tibial slope on mobile-bearing total knee arthroplasty using computational simulation. Knee 2018;25(5):903–14.

21. Lee HY, Kim SJ, Kang KT, et al. The effect of tibial posterior slope on contact force and ligaments stresses in posterior-stabilized total knee arthroplasty-explicit finite element analysis. Knee Surg Relat Res 2012;24(2):91–8.

22. Wang Y, Yan S, Zeng J, et al. The biomechanical effect of different posterior tibial slopes on the tibiofemoral joint after posterior-stabilized total knee arthroplasty. J Orthop Surg 2020;15(1):320.

23. Mullaji AB, Marawar SV, Luthra M. Tibial articular cartilage wear in varus osteoarthritic knees: correlation with anterior cruciate ligament integrity and severity of deformity. J Arthroplasty 2008;23(1):128–35.

24. Moschella D, Blasi A, Leardini A, et al. Wear patterns on tibial plateau from varus osteoarthritic knees. Clin Biomech Bristol Avon 2006;21(2):152–8.

25. Harman MK, Markovich GD, Banks SA, et al. Wear patterns on tibial plateaus from varus and valgus osteoarthritic knees. Clin Orthop 1998;(352): 149–58.

26. Scuderi GR, Kochhar T. Management of flexion contracture in total knee arthroplasty. J Arthroplasty 2007;22(4 Suppl 1):20–4.

27. Holst DC, Doan GW, Angerame MR, et al. What is the effect of posterior osteophytes on flexion and extension gaps in total knee arthroplasty? A cadaveric study. Arthroplasty Today 2021;11:127–33.

28. Kinoshita T, Hino K, Kutsuna T, et al. Efficacy of posterior capsular release for flexion contracture in posterior-stabilized total knee arthroplasty. J Exp Orthop 2021;8(1):102.

29. Campbell TM, Trudel G, Laneuville O. Knee flexion contractures in patients with osteoarthritis: clinical features and histologic characterization of the posterior capsule. Pharm Manag PM R 2015;7(5):466–73.

30. Tibbo ME, Limberg AK, Perry KI, et al. Effect of coronal alignment on 10-year survivorship of a single contemporary total knee arthroplasty. J Clin Med 2021;10(1):142.

31. Matassi F, Pettinari F, Frasconà F, et al. Coronal alignment in total knee arthroplasty: a review. J Orthop Traumatol Off J Ital Soc Orthop Traumatol 2023;24(1):24.

32. Jeremic D. Clinical outcome, postoperative alignment, and implant survivorship after kinematically aligned total knee arthroplasty. In: Howell S, editor. Calipered kinematically aligned total knee arthroplasty [Internet]. Philadelphia, PA: Elsevier; 2022. p. 78–86. Available at: https://linkinghub.elsevier.com/retrieve/pii/B9780323756266000135.

33. Pinskerova V, Vavrik P. Knee anatomy and biomechanics and its relevance to knee replacement. In: Rivière C, Vendittoli PA, editors. Personalized hip and knee joint replacement [Internet]. Cham (CH): Springer; 2020. p. 159–68 [cited 2023 Mar 5]. Available at: http://www.ncbi.nlm.nih.gov/books/NBK565765/.

34. Bottros J, Gad B, Krebs V, et al. Gap balancing in total knee arthroplasty. J Arthroplasty 2006;21(4):11–5.

35. Nowakowski AM, Majewski M, Müller-Gerbl M, et al. Measurement of knee joint gaps without bone resection: "Physiologic" extension and flexion gaps in total knee arthroplasty are asymmetric and unequal and anterior and posterior cruciate ligament resections produce different gap changes. J Orthop Res 2012;30(4):522–7.

36. Victor J. Rotational alignment of the distal femur: a literature review. Orthop Traumatol Surg Res 2009; 95(5):365–72.

37. Ko DO, Lee S, Kim JH, et al. The influence of femoral internal rotation on patellar tracking in total knee arthroplasty using gap technique. Clin Orthop Surg 2021;13(3):352–7.

38. Heesterbeek PJC, Keijsers NLW, Wymenga AB. Femoral component rotation after balanced gap total knee replacement is not a predictor for postoperative patella position. Knee Surg Sports Traumatol Arthrosc 2011;19(7):1131–6.

Troubleshooting Robotics During Total Hip and Knee Arthroplasty

Andreas Fontalis, MD, MSc (Res), MRCS (Eng)[a,b,*],
Shanil Hansjee, BA, BM, BCh[a],
Dia Eldean Giebaly, MBChB, MSc, FRCS (Tr&Orth), MBA[a],
Fabio Mancino, MD[a], Ricci Plastow, MBChB, FRCS (Eng)[a],
Fares S. Haddad, BSc, MD(Res), MCh(Orth), FRCS(Orth), FFSEM[a,b]

KEYWORDS

- Robotic-arm assistance • Troubleshooting • Total hip arthroplasty • Total knee arthroplasty
- Safety • Array

KEY POINTS

- A comprehensive understanding of robotic technology and devices is necessary to overcome potential difficulties and avoid pitfalls.
- If the numbers on the screen do not make sense: failure or suboptimal registration, array loosening, or anatomic reasons are the commonest explanations.
- Potential issues that may be encountered during registration, verification, and pin loosening can normally be pre-empted or rectified by following recovery algorithms.
- There is reassuring evidence to suggest the adoption of robotic technology is safe, and future registry data will be of paramount importance.

 Video content accompanies this article at http://www.orthopedic.theclinics.com.

INTRODUCTION

Advanced technology and complex processing have become ubiquitous in modern life. Appropriate application of technological advances is important in the development of modern medical practice. Although robotics already sees considerable use in other surgical specialties, such as urology, robotic-arm assisted arthroplasty remains a relatively novel field. Given the nature of the procedures and potential consequence of errors, introduction of new technology is often met with apposite examination and understandable concerns; robotic arthroplasty is no exception.

Robotic-arm assistance in arthroplasty was first witnessed in the 1990s with the introduction of the first-generation robotic devices including ROBODOC (THINK Surgical, USA) and CASPER (Universal Robotic Systems Ortho, Germany).[1] Preoperative planning, like modern robotic systems, involved optimization and personalization of implant positioning, following the generation of a 3-dimensional virtual reconstruction of the patient's anatomy. Nevertheless, these systems were "fully active" and while the surgeon was

[a] Department of Trauma and Orthopaedic Surgery, University College Hospital, 235 Euston Road, London, NW1 2BU, UK; [b] Division of Surgery and Interventional Science, University College London, Gower Street, London WC1E 6BT, UK
* Corresponding author. Department of Trauma and Orthopaedic Surgery, University College Hospital, 235 Euston Road, London, NW1 2BU
E-mail address: andreasfontalis@doctors.org.uk
Twitter: @AFontalis (A.F.)

Orthop Clin N Am 55 (2024) 33–48
https://doi.org/10.1016/j.ocl.2023.06.004
0030-5898/24/© 2023 Elsevier Inc. All rights reserved.

involved in the preoperative planning phase, there was limited input intraoperatively confined to an emergency stop. These first-generation fully active robotic systems were linked to higher complication rates, including inadvertent soft tissue damage, femoral fractures, and high conversion rates to manual procedure.[1–3] Conceivably, this perpetuated skepticism among arthroplasty surgeons concerning the adoption of this new technology. Owing to the increased risk of complications and litigation issues, the above systems are no longer used in modern orthopedic practice.

The evolution of surgical technology, however, resulted in the advent of semiactive robotic systems, which unlike their predecessors, are not fully automated. They are effectively surgical slaves allowing the surgeon to maintain overall control of the tibial and femoral cuts, acetabular reaming, alignment, and implant positioning.[4] Hence, the surgeon's role is vital with the robotic-arm simply delivering a surgeon's devised plan.

This article focuses on providing a general understanding and stepwise approach on the introduction of new technology in surgery and presents comprehensive solutions and troubleshooting workflows for robotic-arm assisted total hip arthroplasty (THA) and total knee arthroplasty (TKA). To this end, the article also incorporates the available evidence regarding intraoperative complications with robotic technology.

HISTORY
Lessons Learnt in Orthopedic Surgery from the Introduction of Navigation
By examining the introduction of various technologies in the field of surgery, it becomes evident that many of the challenges encountered can be overcome through a comprehensive understanding of the new operative procedures and troubleshooting techniques.

Arguably, one of the most transformative advancements in contemporary arthroplasty practice is the emergence of computer assisted orthopedic surgery. The initial reports documenting the development of the first computerized tomography (CT)-based navigation system were published by DiGioia et al in Pittsburgh in 1994,[5] where computer guidance was employed to position the acetabular cup.

At the core of every robotic or navigation system lies a navigator. Its primary function is to establish a 3-dimensional coordinate system and facilitate the exchange of positional data among the patient, surgical instruments, and the surgeon.[6] Robotic systems inherently encompass the role of the navigator within the robot itself, whereas surgical navigation employs a position tracking device. Real-time positional feedback for bony resection is enabled through the utilization of infrared or electromagnetic registration signaling.[7–9]

In surgical procedures using navigation technology, the surgeon is required to insert temporary pins either intraincisionally or through separate stab incisions. In hip arthroplasty procedures, pins are secured in the ilium, whereas knee arthroplasty navigation involves the insertion of pins in the femoral and tibial diaphysis. Although the pins are generally considered innocuous, they represent an additional procedural step and could conceptually lead to complications such as pin-related fractures, infection, or soft tissue injury. Initially, these concerns instilled skepticism amongst early adopters.[10] However, extensive research conducted over several years has not substantiated the apprehension of increased complication rates.

In one of the largest studies conducted in the United States, analysis of the American College of Surgeons National Surgical Quality Improvement Program database (NSQIP) revealed a lower risk of medical morbidity in patients undergoing navigated TKA compared with conventional procedures, primarily attributed to a reduced risk of blood transfusion.[11] Furthermore, no significant differences were observed in operative time, length of stay, and readmission, thereby affirming the safety of navigation.[11] Moreover, large-scale studies have reported the incidence of fractures associated with pins as low as 0.065%.[12] A recent systematic review encompassing 36 studies on the safety of computer-assisted navigation and robotic-arm assistance revealed a low occurrence of pin-related complications, with the most common being pin dislodgement (0.6%) and superficial pin site infections (0.6%), further consolidating the body of evidence supporting their safety.[13]

Additionally, it is crucial to recognize that the current robotic systems are the outcome of extensive development and evolution, resulting in clinically robust technology that complies with rigorous regulations. Furthermore, considering the technology adoption lifecycle (innovators, early adopters, early majority, late majority, and laggard),[14] computer-assisted arthroplasty surgery has advanced beyond the initial phases. Consequently, appropriate support and training resources are now readily available.

BACKGROUND

The FDA data presented by Almezadeh and colleagues[15] on the outcomes of minimally invasive surgery indicate that new technologies are not without risks; a non-negligible number of complications occur. It is therefore all the more important to recognize these potential hazards and consider methods by which to negate them and minimize patient morbidity.

As robotic arthroplasty has advanced, there here has been an increase in the available platforms. It is important to distinguish the type of system used to understand the possible issues and solutions one might encounter. Available robotic-arm assisted arthroplasty platforms can be divided into image-based and image-free systems. Further delineation of these devices is outlined below.

Of the current robotic systems in primary TKA (Table 1), the TSolution One (THINK Surgical, USA) is the only fully active robotic system on the market.[16] It provides a fully automatic option, with resection from a preoperative plan, after correlation with intraoperative bone mapping. Furthermore, it is the only system encompassing an open platform, offering inter-brand compatibility in relation to implant choice. Because of the automation, TSolution One is less adaptable intraoperatively than the other leading systems.

The MAKO SmartRobotics Robotic Arm Interactive Orthopedic system (Stryker Corp, Mako Surgical Corp, Ft. Lauderdale, FL, USA) is a semi-active robotic system and together with TSolution One require a preoperative CT to create a 3-dimensional plan of the patient's anatomy and customize implant positioning. This is subsequently combined with additional intraoperative mapping that creates a navigated map of the knee, surface matched to the CT scan. Although this comes at the cost of additional imaging, processing, and radiation exposure, it has the potential benefits of additional precision and protection from intraoperative error. The ROSA Knee system (Zimmer-Biomet, Warsaw, IN, USA) also has the capacity to function as an image-based system, with the use of X-ray guidance. Image-free robotic systems functioning solely on intraoperative mapping include the CORI Surgical System (Smith & Nephew, Watford, UK), a handheld semi-active robotic system; OMNI-Botics (Corin, Circencester, UK), a jig-based robotic system anchoring to the patient's knee; and the VELYS Robotic-assisted Solution (DePuy Synthes, Rayham, MA, USA), a semi-active robotic system that has received FDA approval in the United States but is not yet licensed outside North America.[16]

As a consequence of its automation, TSolution One is also the only system that does not incorporate dynamic data. Measurements with the semi-active systems are recorded using varus and valgus stress through a range of motion enabling a virtual representation of the soft tissue knee envelope. All systems benefit from designated product specialists for console operation and assistance. The CORI and ROSA products additionally have a touchscreen that can be draped to enable surgeon interaction. The visual output and graphical data displays vary from product to product.

To ensure accuracy, ROSA aids the surgeon with the application of cutting jigs and bone preparation is then performed manually. The other systems use a burr or saw, confounded by the boundaries set from the virtual 3D model. Although MAKO uses a saw or burr, mounted on a robotic arm capable of providing haptic feedback, CORI uses a smart burr that stops or retracts if the operating surgeon strays beyond the predetermined boundaries. TSolution One aims to improve accuracy through physical fixation of femur and tibia to the robot.

With the exception of MAKO, which is used both in hip and knee arthroplasty, the other devices are currently joint specific. Notwithstanding this, robotic systems are subject to similar hazards as they share the same principles governing robotic-arm assisted arthroplasty.

MAKO is currently the most commonly used robotic system in THA worldwide.[17] MAKO THA is CT-based and following the generation of a patient specific plan, the robotic system provides audio-visual and haptic feedback to guide acetabular reaming and cup positioning within predefined stereotactic boundaries.[1] Other commercially available systems include the ROSA system (Zimmer-Biomet, Warsaw, IN) that uses preoperative radiographs for surgical planning. Of note, it is solely used for the direct anterior approach and uses intraoperative fluoroscopic guidance instead of preoperative CT or navigation pins.[17] Furthermore, other companies that offer robotic-arm assisted TKA have launched hip navigation platforms including the VELYS Hip Navigation platform (DePuy Synthes, Rayham, MA, USA), and CORI RI.HIP NAVIGATION and RI.HIP MODELER (Smith & Nephew, Watford, UK).

Troubleshooting Robotics

The common underlying themes for early adoption of new surgical tools include technical

Table 1
Summary of characteristics among available robotic systems in primary total knee arthroplasty

Name and Company of the Robotic Device	THINK Surgical TSolution One	Stryker MAKO	Zimmer Biomet Rosa	Smith and Nephew CORI	Corin OMNIbotics	Depuy Velys
Process	Automatic	Collaborative	Collaborative	Collaborative	Collaborative	Collaborative
Image based?	CT scan	CT scan	X-Atlas™ (X-ray)/Imageless	Imageless	Imageless	Imageless
Dynamic data	Not used	Extension and 90°	Dynamic assessment	Dynamic assessment	Dynamic assessment	Dynamic assessment
Bone preparation	Automated robotic preparation of bone (preplanned) with surgeon protecting soft tissue	Robotic arm mounted saw/burr with haptic feedback	Robotic positioning of cutting jig Manual bone preparation	Smart burr deactivates/retracts when outside of planned margins	Robotic positioning of femoral cutting guide and confirmation of tibial guide orientation	Arm mounted saw with deactivation when outside planned boundaries

Table 2
Issues that might occur with image-based or image-free robotic systems at different stages and troubleshooting solutions

Stage	Problems	Troubleshooting Solutions
Preoperative planning stage	Inadequate CT planning (image-based systems)	• Imaging protocol not followed, field of view or slice thickness incorrect: use raw imaging data • Motion detection: field of view reduction to encapsulate the minimum required anatomy that is salvageable • CT scan not reconstructible: repeat CT scan

Registration	Checkpoint verification unsuccessful following registration	• Go back to bone registration or mapping
		  ○ Bony registration successful in all 3 planes ➡ checkpoint has moved
		  ○ Clear checkpoint, remove, re-insert into hard bone and re-capture
		• Go back to bone registration or mapping
		  ○ Bone registration in either of the 3 planes fails or registration error unacceptable ➡ array has moved
		  ○ Clear bone registration and landmarks
		  ○ Tighten the array
		  ○ Re-register bone

Bone cuts	Inability to verify the sawblade or cutting guide checkpoint prior to performing the bone cuts	• Incorrect assembly of the saw
		  ○ Correct saw attachment, saw blade, or cutting guide used
		  ○ Firmly tightened
		• If the above fails ➡ array has likely moved
		  ○ Tighten the base array and re-register
		• If the checkpoint has moved ➡ follow the recovery workflow described above (registration phase)

Any stage	Pin loosening	• Before cuts
		  ○ Reposition pins or use more pins (3-pin pelvis array in robotic THA)
		  ○ Re-register
		• After cuts in robotic TKA or UKA

(continued on next page)

Table 2 (continued)		
Stage	**Problems**	**Troubleshooting Solutions**
		o If bone still present in the transverse plane: re-register (see Fig. 5) o Minimum one verification mark is necessary o Re-register with lateral tibia in UKA • If all above fails ➡ convert to manual procedure

Any stage	Bumped array	• Knocked before cuts
		  o Re-register
		• Knocked after some cuts made
		  o Recover previous position, tighten the array and verify
		  o If unsuccessful ➡ repeat registration: tighten the array, clear bone registration, checkpoints and landmarks and re-capture
		• Knocked after reaming in express workflow robotic THA
		  o Manual impaction of the cup
		  o Final inclination and anteversion can be checked
		  o Final position can be re-adjusted (with cementless cups)

experience and operator comfort. This cannot be achieved without first considering the potential pitfalls and techniques to overcome them. The common issues among the different image-based and image-free robotic devices that can occur during robotic-arm assisted THA and TKA are illustrated in Tables 2 and 3. Furthermore, troubleshooting solutions and technical tips tailored to the individual robotic system are also discussed.

Preoperative Planning Stage

In some circumstances the preoperative planning with image-based robotic systems may be inadequate. This showcases the importance of performing the CT as early as possible, to allow ample time to promptly identify and pre-empt potential problems. However, it should be taken into consideration that acquisition of the CT is not recommended earlier than 6 months prior to the procedure.

Errors can be rectified by re-constructing the CT, and specific solutions are presented below. If the imaging protocol has not been followed and the field of view or slice thickness is incorrect, the raw data can be used to reduce the field of view. If motion is detected, then a reduction in the field of view can be attempted to only have the minimum required anatomy that can be salvaged. Effective communication is key, as the majority of scans will be salvageable, or else the scan may need repeating.

Registration

A principal concern with robotic technology surrounds the registration phase (Fig. 1, Video 1) and available solutions if the registration error is too large or it fails. At the end of the registration phase, there is a verification result, reflecting the accuracy to the 3D CT model (Fig. 2A, B) and this is really important for the surgeon to note. If later on the numbers do not make

Table 3 Useful technical tips to avoid pitfalls	
Stage	**Troubleshooting Solutions**
Preoperative planning stage	Perform CT as early as possible, generally no earlier than 6 mo prior to the procedure (image-based systems)
Registration	Adequate exposure, retraction, optimal utilization of assistants to access posterior condyle for mapping (key in image-free systems) Checkpoints in hard bone and approximately 10 mm from the projected bone cuts Array connections aligned properly, engaging the apposed serrations Adjust camera to ensure all tracking arrays are visible throughout the full ROM Avoid areas of osteophytes
Robotic THA	Carefully consider the ergonomics and set up of the operating room Most common reasons for array loosening/movement are impaction of the robotic device on the bed or reamer on the robot
Pin placement	Carefully consider bone quality In soft bone, key to achieve bicortical pin placement Ideally in the femoral diaphysis and not the metaphysis Robotic THA: could use a 3-pin pelvic array Avoid multiple attempts
Bone cuts	Technical tip to avoid spillage on the array discs Cover the array not in use with a surgical gauze (eg, the tibia array when femoral cutis performed)

sense, it could potentially be traced back to not having achieved the desired accuracy. Hence, there may be a need to repeat the registration (see Table 2).

The surgeon has to ensure trackers are visible, in the event the respective error appears during the registration phase (Fig. 3). Should there be movement of the robotic unit or camera, the registration will fail. Hence, it should be verified

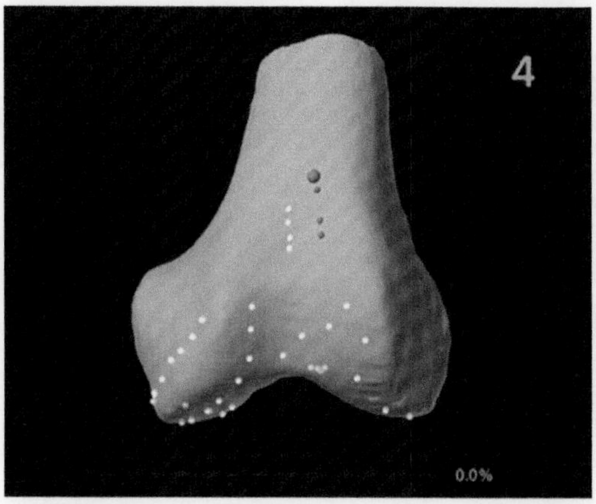

Fig. 1. Registration with an image-based robotic system (MAKO).

that the robotic (each wheel and the main immobilization system) and optical units are immobilized. Furthermore, registration issues can be eluded by ensuring the appropriate tightening of the arrays and reference frames that should be fully seated and tight on the instruments (Video 2).

Should checkpoint verification be unsuccessful following registration in image-based systems; technical issues can be broken down into problems with movement of the checkpoint or the array. For the arthroplasty surgeon to ascertain the etiology, it is necessary to go back to the bony registration. If bony registration is successful in all 3 planes; the issue is likely related to checkpoint movement, which should be cleared, removed, re-inserted into hard bone and re-captured (see Table 2). As a rule of thumb, checkpoints should be placed in hard bone and located approximately 10 mm from the projected bone cuts. Occasionally, surgeons may choose to use alternative landmarks or anatomic points as checkpoints; however, it is beyond the scope of this article to investigate the validity and accuracy of this approach.

In case the bone registration in any of the 3 planes fails or the registration error is

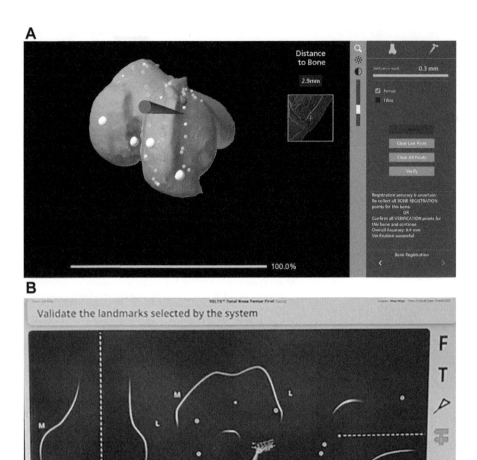

Fig. 2. (*A, B*) The registration verification in image-based and image-free systems.

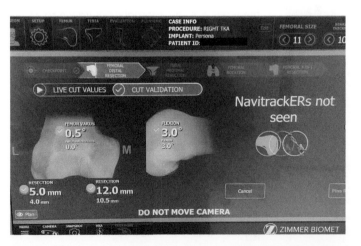

Fig. 3. The screen error when trackers are not seen in ROSA robotic system.

unacceptable, the array has likely moved. This scenario mandates clearing the bone registration and landmarks, tightening the array and re-executing the entire bone registration. Users should ensure the connections within the array assembly are aligned properly, engaging the apposed serrations to prevent loss of bone registration during the case (see Video 2). Further useful points include ensuring the camera is adjusted such that all tracking arrays are visible from full extension to full flexion and when walking bone during registration; areas of osteophytes are avoided, as they can produce erroneous results on the screen.

With image-free systems, such as CORI and VELYS, it is essential to achieve accurate mapping. A challenging technical aspect that can be encountered when mapping is access to the posterior condyle. Therefore, adequate exposure and retraction as well as optimal utilization of assistants is critical at this stage.

Verification of the Sawblade or Cutting Guide Checkpoint

One of the more common issues seen during robotic workflow, is the inability to verify the sawblade or cutting guide checkpoint prior to performing the bone cuts; the most common cause being incorrect assembly of the saw. Hence, it should be verified the correct saw attachment (angled vs sagittal in MAKO), saw blade (narrow vs standard) or cutting guide (Persona, NexGen, Vanguard in ROSA), and laterality (A or B) are used. Moreover, the cutting guide should be firmly tightened and the discs on the base array should also be checked. In THA cases using MAKO, more assembly checks of the reamer and impactor can be performed especially if the offset reamer is used.

If all above techniques fail, it should be assumed the base array/reference frame has moved, in which case it needs to be tightened and the registration process repeated. In robotic THA, movement of the base array can occur if the robotic arm is knocked against the bed or the reamer knocks against the robot, highlighting the importance of carefully planning the operating room set up and ergonomics.

Array Knocked or Moved

One of the dominant concerns among users of robotic systems in arthroplasty is troubleshooting options if the array is knocked or moved during the procedure. Globally recognized standards, such as those published by the ASTM (American Society for Testing and Materials), exist to ensure the robustness and accuracy of mounted arrays.

The ASTM's F3107 to 14(2023) standard, for example, aims to measure the effect of vibrations caused by cutting saws, burrs, drills, and impact loading on the accuracy of robotic systems in a reproducible manner. Robotic manufacturers should adhere to similar standards to establish appropriate safety.[18]

In the event of array movement, the registration needs to be repeated. Notwithstanding this, a bigger problem is posed if some but not all cuts have been made. In this scenario, the use of an image-based robotic system confers an advantage as there is a model the surgeon can revisit. If the array moves after some cuts have been made, every effort should be made to recover the previous position, tighten the array, and verify according to the checkpoint (Fig. 4). As long as points in 3 planes are verified, it is possible to proceed with caution and after walking the bone with the probe to ensure the 3D model is correct.

In the scenario where the previous position of the array cannot be recovered, the registration needs to be repeated. The recovery workflow includes in sequence, tightening of the array, clearing the bone registration, checkpoints, and landmarks and recapturing them. When re-registering the bone, it is prudent to avoid sites of osteophyte removal or where cuts have already been made. For example, in cases where a cruciate retaining (CR) implant is used, the uncut edge of the posterior medial tibia can be used to re-register (Fig. 5).

Pins loosen vary rarely and if this happens, the course of action depends on the stage of the procedure. If pins become loose before the cuts are made, they can be repositioned or more pins can be used (use 3-pin pelvis array in robotic THA). In the scenario where pins move after the cuts in robotic TKA; if bone is still present in the transverse plane, re-registration can be performed and as a minimum only one verification mark is necessary (see Fig. 5). In robotic unicompartmental knee arthroplasty (UKA), re-registration can be performed with the lateral tibia. Ultimately if all the above fails, there may be a need to convert to manual procedure; although the probability of this occurrence is very rare.

With respect to the express workflow in robotic THA using MAKO, if the pelvic array moves after reaming, the cup will have to be impacted manually. However, the final inclination and anteversion can be checked, which offers the opportunity to still change the acetabular cup orientation if a cementless cup is used.

Bone quality is an important consideration and pre-emptive measures should be taken

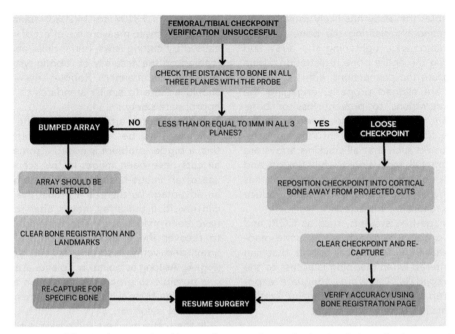

Fig. 4. Recovery workflow in the scenario of bumped array or loose checkpoint during robotic-arm assisted TKA and THA.

to avoid complications in osteoporotic patients. In soft bone, it is key to achieve bicortical pin placement and ideally, they should be positioned in the femoral diaphysis and not the metaphysis. In robotic THA, another option is to use more pins and use a 3-pin pelvic array.

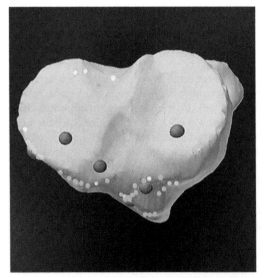

Fig. 5. Verification marks during robotic-arm assisted TKA. In this case, bone was registered using the uncut edge of the posterior medial tibia in a CR knee.

Malfunctioning of the Robotic Device, Arm, or Handpiece

There may be occasions, albeit very rare, where the equipment fails or there is unexpected malfunction of the system. Should problems with moving the robotic device be encountered, the foot pedal should be checked. If broken, it can be manually lifted (Fig. 6). With the MAKO system, if the robotic arm locks while cutting or reaming, this is likely secondary to excessive force. The product specialist will have to put a safety stop on and release the arm manually to override the system. The surgeon will then have to physically remove or pull the arm of the robot (approximately 30 kg) (Fig. 7).

If the robotic arm of the ROSA system drifts slowly in collaborative mode, or the movement of the robotic arm is interrupted, an unsuitable tool has likely been installed. This can be resolved by installing the corresponding tool to the current stage of the procedure and restarting movement.

With the CORI system, should the robotic-controlled handpiece stop working, it should be re-assembled as it may not have been screwed in properly. It should be ensured that the burr retracts appropriately and if issues persist, the handpiece can be changed.

A very useful technical tip to avoid spillage on the array discs and subsequently malfunctioning during the bone cuts in robotic TKA with any

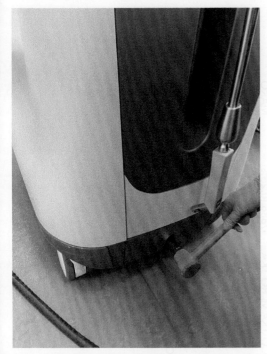

Fig. 6. Troubleshooting in case issues with movement of the robotic device is encountered.

system is to cover the array not in use with a surgical gauze (eg, the tibial array when femoral cuts are performed).

OUTCOMES AND SAFETY PROFILE OF SEMI-ACTIVE SYSTEMS

Despite very few studies designed to specifically study intra-operative complications with robotic technology as a primary outcome, available evidence is reassuring and suggests a very low incidence of intraoperative problems and pin

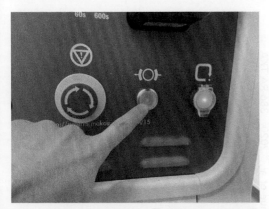

Fig. 7. The manual override of the MAKO robotic system in case the robotic arm needs to be released.

related complications during robotic-arm assisted THA and TKA.

Vermue and colleagues[19] retrospectively reviewed all robotic-arm assisted TKAs between April 2018 and September 2019 following the introduction of the MAKO robotic platform (N = 386). Patients who underwent conventional TKA surgery prior to the introduction of the surgical robot were included as a control group (N = 263). Femoral pins were positioned in the wound underneath the vastus medialis and tibial pins 10 cm below the surgical incision. Authors reported only one complication related to tibial pin placement owing to suboptimal positioning, causing a diaphyseal stress fracture that healed uneventfully after 8 weeks.

Another study that highlights the very rare incidence of pin loosening and intraoperative complications with robotic technology was performed by Yun and colleagues[20] (N = 2603 knees) who used a unicortical technique for pin placement in robotic UKA and TKA using the MAKO robot. In the bicortical diaphyseal group, femoral shaft fractures occurred in 3 of 1571 (0.19%) limbs within the first 3 months after surgery and were caused by minor or no visible trauma. The fracture sites lay at the femoral array pin hole. Conversely, no fracture was reported in the unicortical periarticular group. No array loosening was observed in either group. The authors advocated for the use of unicortical periarticular pin placement in computer-navigated and robotic-arm assisted knee arthroplasty. Conversely, excessive movement of the array may be encountered when using unicortical pins and should be avoided in osteoporotic bone.

Smith and colleagues[21] reported no fractures or postoperative revisions when comparing a total of 120 consecutive patients undergoing RO-TKA with a prospective cohort of 103 consecutive patients undergoing CO TKA with manual jig-based instruments during the same time period. Furthermore, Kayani and colleagues[22] in a prospective cohort study comparing 40 RO TKAs with 40 CO TKAs reported only one case of wound dehiscence in each group, successfully treated with antibiotics.

Held and colleagues[23] in their retrospective review encompassing 111 consecutive robotic-arm assisted TKAs using the NAVIO imageless surgical system and 111 consecutive conventional TKAs reported the total number of patients who experienced a postoperative complication or reoperation was comparable. One case of patella tendon rupture was encountered in each group and one patient (0.9%) in the robotic cohort required reoperation for

Table 4
Summary of studies and complications related to robotic-arm assisted knee arthroplasty with semi-active systems

Author, Date and Evidence Level	Sample Size	Methodological Features	Outcomes	Controls	Key Results	Robotic Device or Implants Used
Yun et al,[20] 2021 Level III	1702 RO TKA 901 RO UKA	Retrospective review Single center (3 senior surgeons) June 2017- December 2019 Minimum 1 y follow-up	Complications, periprosthetic fractures, revision surgery Array loosening requiring abortion of the robotic-arm assisted procedure	Unicortical pin (UP) placement vs bicortical pin placement (BP)	0.19% femoral shaft fractures in BP group, no fractures in the UP group No array loosening in either group	MAKO Triathlon for TKA Restoris MCK for UKA
Kayani et al,[22] 2018 Level II	40 RO TKA 40 CO TKA	Single center Prospective data collection Single Surgeon	Postoperative pain Postoperative hemoglobin Functional outcomes 30-d complication rate Length of stay	CO TKA vs RO TKA	1 minor wound dehiscence in each group	MAKO cemented Triathlon PS
Vermue et al,[19] 2020 Level III	386 RA TKA 263 CO TKA	Retrospective review Single center 6 surgeons	Operative times Implant and limb alignment Intraoperative joint balance Robot-related complications	CO TKA vs RO TKA	1/386 (0.26%) diaphyseal tibial stress fracture (related to the tibial pin placement)	MAKO Triathlon
Smith et al,[21] 2019 Level III	120 RA TKA 103 CO TKA	Retrospective review of consecutive patients 12 mo follow-up	KSS Likert Scoring LOS; Operation time Complications	CO TKA vs RO TKA	9 MUAs in both groups No fractures or revision	MAKO Triathlon

Held et al,[23] 2022 Level III	111 RO TKA 110 CO TKA	Retrospective cohort analysis Multi surgeon 24 mo follow-up	PROMs (KSS-FS; WOMAC; SF-12) Surgical complications ROM Operative time Estimated blood loss	CO TKA vs RO TKA	Patellar tendon rupture 1/111 in RO group (0.9%) vs 1/110 in CO group (0.9%) 1 tibial fracture from pin site (0.9%) in RO TKA group vs no fracture in CO TKA group	NAVIO Journey II BCS
Vanlommel et al,[24] 2021 Level III	90 imageless RO TKA 90 CO TKA	Retrospective cohort 3 high volume surgeons Single center Minimum 3 mo follow-up	Learning curve Operative time Accuracy of achieving planned alignment Complications	CO TKA vs RO TKA	No intraoperative or postoperative complications	ROSA
Thomas et al,[13] 2022 Level I	18 case reports (25 cases) 18 RCTs (7336 cases)	Systematic review	Incidence, timing, treatment, and clinical outcomes of tracking pin-related Complications following CN and Robotic-arm assisted knee arthroplasty	N/A	Overall pin-related complications rate 1.4% Most common: pin dislodgement (0.6%) and superficial pin site infections (0.6%) Most postoperative complications at the tibial site (69%)	All systems

Abbreviations: CN, computer navigation; CO TKA, conventional TKA; KSS, Knee Society Clinical Rating System; LOS, length of stay; MUA, manipulation under anesthesia; PROMs, patient reported outcome measures; RCT, randomized controlled trial; RO TKA, robotic-arm assisted TKA; ROM, range of motion; WOMAC, Western Ontario and McMaster Universities Arthritis Index.

periprosthetic distal femoral shaft fracture secondary to a fall. The number of surgical site complications did not differ significantly between the 2 cohorts. Of note, among the 10 superficial wound complications in the RO-TKA group, 3 involved the pin sites. One unicortical tibial shaft stress fracture at the pin site was reported in the RO-TKA group, which was minimally displaced and managed nonoperatively. This healed uneventfully without modification of the normal postoperative weight-bearing protocol.

Vanlommel and colleagues[24] in their retrospective cohort study comparing the results of 90 RO-TKA (ROSA knee system, Zimmer Biomet, Montreal, Quebec, Canada) versus 90 manual CO TKA cases reported no intraoperative or postoperative complications associated with the robotic system. Postoperative complications were rare and included arthrofibrosis (2 RO TKA vs 1 CO TKA), surgical site infections (RO TKA = 1, CO TKA = 3), deep vein thrombosis (RO-TKA = 1, CO TKA = 0), and periprosthetic joint infection (RO TKA = 0, CO TKA = 1).

One of the rare complications seen with robotic TKA, with a reassuringly low incidence in the literature, is femoral or tibial shaft fractures due to mechanical weakness caused by the pinholes. Yun and colleagues[20] recommended periarticular pin placement as the bone at this site is more robust to torsional and bending stresses than the diaphysis, whereas Vermue and colleagues[19] advocated for smaller pins to prevent this complication. Pin-site infection is another specific complication of the tracker pin that may require antibiotics and dressing for an additional duration. However, the incidence has generally been reported to be low (0.47%).[23]

What constitutes likely the highest-level evidence regarding complications with navigation and robotic technology to date is a recently published systematic review encompassing 36 studies. Authors reported an overall rate of pin-related complications of 1.4%; with pin dislodgment (0.6%) and superficial pin site infections (0.6%) quoted as the most common. Most complications occurred at the tibia site and had resolved during follow-up.[13] Of note, most primary studies in this systematic review comprised computer navigation. It should be considered that despite sharing similar principles to pin placement during robotic-arm assistance, the safety profile may differ (Table 4).

SUMMARY

Robotic-arm assistance is a valuable tool in the surgical armamentarium and has been associated with improved accuracy of implant positioning[25] and reduced soft tissue injury,[26,27] while data pertaining to improvements in functional and patient reported outcomes have been inconclusive to date.[17]

The introduction of any new technology mandates advanced understanding of the new technology and troubleshooting strategies to prevent potential errors during surgery. Most complications in robotic THA and TKA occur as part of the learning curve, which does not appear to be associated with achieving the desired accuracy or precision.[28] It is about integration into the surgical workflow, streamlining parts of the operation, improving surgical confidence and comfort of the surgical team. In this vein, it has been suggested that previous experience with navigation or the presence of a surgeon experienced in robotic arthroplasty flattens the curve and is likely to help in averting complications.[29]

It is possible with any available robotic devices on the market that they malfunction. However, based on published evidence, this is extremely rare and most devices have redundancies built in. Patient safety will always be of paramount importance when introducing new technology in surgery and the troubleshooting workflows mentioned in this article along with technical support and manual instrumentation are essential to preventing complications.

One of the most challenging scenarios is identifying the issue if the numbers on the robotic screen do not make sense. In that event, situational awareness of the arthroplasty surgeon is vital. The problem is commonly related to failure or suboptimal registration, loosening of the array or may pertain to anatomic reasons and the way robotic technology functions. For example, the knee fixed flexion angle displayed with robotics and navigation depends on the bow of the femur and anteversion of the femoral neck and may not entirely correlate with what is evident clinically, something that the surgeon may need to mentally adjust for.

There is reassuring evidence to date suggesting the occurrence of robotic system-specific complications is rare and the adoption of this technology is safe. Data pertaining to complications and outcomes following robotic-arm assisted arthroplasty are not currently included in registries of the United States, Canada, Australia, or the United Kingdom and future registry data will be valuable to further evaluate the safety profile of robotic technology. Furthermore, with the ever-growing number of companies and robotic devices on the market it is of paramount importance to generate high-quality evidence for each system separately.

CLINICS CARE POINTS

- As showcased by the introduction of other technologies in surgery, such as navigation, it becomes apparent that concerns faced could be overcome when acquiring a more comprehensive understanding of the technology, potential pitfalls, and available strategies to overcome them.

- In some circumstances preoperative planning may be inadequate; hence, it is helpful to perform the CT as early as possible. Potential solutions if the CT protocol has not been followed include using the raw data or reducing the field of view.

- If the array is bumped after some cuts have been made, every attempt should be made to recover the previous position and if not feasible; the array should be tightened, bone registration, checkpoints, and landmarks cleared and re-captured.

- If the numbers do not make sense, situational awareness is of paramount importance. Failure or suboptimal registration, loosening of the array or anatomic reasons should be considered (eg, parameters that can create disparity between the clinical fixed flexion and display on the screen).

DISCLOSURE

F.S. Haddad reports the following: Journal of Bone and Joint Surgery–British: Board of membership. Royalties: Smith & Nephew, Corin, MatOrtho and Stryker. Payment for lectures including service on speakers' bureaus: Smith & Nephew, and Stryker, United States. Paid consultant; Research support; Stryker.

ACKNOWLEDGMENT

Andreas Fontalis would like to thank the Onassis Foundation for the financial support of his PhD studies - Scholarship ID: F ZR 065-1/ 2021-2022.

SUPPLEMENTARY DATA

Supplementary data related to this article can be found online at https://doi.org/10.1016/j.ocl.2023.06.004.

REFERENCES

1. Fontalis A, Kayani B, Thompson JW, et al. Robotic total hip arthroplasty: past, present and future. Orthop Trauma 2022;36(1):6–13.
2. Mart JPS, Goh EL, Shah Z. Robotics in total hip arthroplasty: a review of the evolution, application and evidence base. EFORT Open Rev 2020;5(12): 866.
3. Han P-F, Chen C-L, Zhang Z-L, et al. Robotics-assisted versus conventional manual approaches for total hip arthroplasty: A systematic review and meta-analysis of comparative studies. Int J Med Robot 2019;15(3). https://doi.org/10.1002/RCS.1990.
4. Fontalis A, Epinette JA, Thaler M, et al. Advances and innovations in total hip arthroplasty. SICOT J 2021;7. https://doi.org/10.1051/SICOTJ/2021025.
5. Digioia A.M., Simon D.A., Jaramaz B., et al., Hip-Nav: pre-operative planning and intra-operative navigational guidance for acetabular implant placement in total hip replacement surgery. In Proc CAOS Symp., Bern, 1995.
6. Zheng G, Nolte LP. Computer-Assisted Orthopedic Surgery: Current State and Future Perspective. Front Surg 2015;2:66.
7. Lionberger DR, Weise J, Ho DM, et al. How Does Electromagnetic Navigation Stack Up Against Infrared Navigation in Minimally Invasive Total Knee Arthroplasties? J Arthroplasty 2008;23(4):573–80.
8. Stulberg DD, Picard F, Saragaglia D. Computer-assisted total knee replacement arthroplasty. Oper Tech Orthop 2000;10(1):25–39.
9. Lionberger DR. The attraction of electromagnetic computer-assisted navigation in orthopaedic surgery. Navigation and MIS in Orthopaedic Surgery 2007;44–53.
10. Picard F, Deakin AH, Riches PE, et al. Computer assisted orthopaedic surgery: past, present and future. Med Eng Phys 2019;72:55–65.
11. Webb ML, Hutchison CE, Sloan M, et al. Reduced postoperative morbidity in computer-navigated total knee arthroplasty: A retrospective comparison of 225,123 cases. Knee 2021;30:148–56.
12. Brown MJ, Matthews JR, Bayers-Thering MT, et al. Low Incidence of Postoperative Complications With Navigated Total Knee Arthroplasty. J Arthroplasty 2017;32(7):2120–6.
13. Thomas TL, Goh GS, Nguyen MK, et al. Pin-Related Complications in Computer Navigated and Robotic-Assisted Knee Arthroplasty: A Systematic Review. J Arthroplasty 2022;37(11):2291–307.e2.
14. Beal GM, Bohlen JM, Coleman L, et al. THE DIFFUSION PROCESS 1956;111–21.
15. Alemzadeh H, Raman J, Leveson N, et al. Adverse Events in Robotic Surgery: A Retrospective Study of 14 Years of FDA Data. PLoS One 2016;11(4). https://doi.org/10.1371/JOURNAL.PONE.0151470.

16. Walgrave S, Oussedik S. Comparative assessment of current robotic-assisted systems in primary total knee arthroplasty. Bone Jt Open 2023;4(1):13–8.

17. Bullock EKC, Brown MJ, Clark G, et al. Robotics in Total Hip Arthroplasty: Current Concepts. J Clin Med 2022;11(22). https://doi.org/10.3390/JCM11226674.

18. F3107 Standard Test Method for Measuring Accuracy After Mechanical Disturbances on Reference Frames of Computer Assisted Surgery Systems. Available at: https://www.astm.org/f3107-14r23.html. Accessed May 12, 2023.

19. Vermue H, Luyckx T, Winnock de Grave P, et al. Robot-assisted total knee arthroplasty is associated with a learning curve for surgical time but not for component alignment, limb alignment and gap balancing. Knee Surg Sports Traumatol Arthrosc 2022;30(2):593–602.

20. Yun AG, Qutami M, Pasko KBD. Do bicortical diaphyseal array pins create the risk of periprosthetic fracture in robotic-assisted knee arthroplasties? Arthroplasty 2021;3(1):1–7.

21. Smith AF, Eccles CJ, Bhimani SJ, et al. Improved Patient Satisfaction following Robotic-Assisted Total Knee Arthroplasty. J Knee Surg 2021;34(7):730–8.

22. Kayani B, Konan S, Pietrzak JRT, et al. Robotic-arm assisted total knee arthroplasty is associated with improved early functional recovery and reduced time to hospital discharge compared with conventional jig-based total knee arthroplasty. Bone and Joint Journal 2018;100B(7):930–7.

23. Held MB, Gazgalis A, Neuwirth AL, et al. Imageless robotic-assisted total knee arthroplasty leads to similar 24-month WOMAC scores as compared to conventional total knee arthroplasty: a retrospective cohort study. Knee Surg Sports Traumatol Arthrosc 2022;30(8):2631–8.

24. Vanlommel L, Neven E, Anderson MB, et al. The initial learning curve for the ROSA® Knee System can be achieved in 6-11 cases for operative time and has similar 90-day complication rates with improved implant alignment compared to manual instrumentation in total knee arthroplasty. J Exp Orthop 2021;8(1). https://doi.org/10.1186/S40634-021-00438-8.

25. Fontalis A, Putzeys P, Plastow R, et al. Functional component positioning in total hip arthroplasty and the role of robotic-arm assistance in addressing spinopelvic pathology. Orthop Clin North Am 2023. https://doi.org/10.1016/J.OCL.2022.11.003.

26. Fontalis A, Kayani B, Asokan A, et al. Inflammatory Response in Robotic-Arm-Assisted Versus Conventional Jig-Based TKA and the Correlation with Early Functional Outcomes: Results of a Prospective Randomized Controlled Trial. J Bone Joint Surg Am 2022;104(21):1905–14.

27. Kayani B, Tahmassebi J, Ayuob A, et al. A prospective randomized controlled trial comparing the systemic inflammatory response in conventional jig-based total knee arthroplasty versus robotic-arm assisted total knee arthroplasty. Bone Joint Lett J 2021;103-B(1):113–22.

28. Kayani B, Konan S, Huq SS, et al. Robotic-arm assisted total knee arthroplasty has a learning curve of seven cases for integration into the surgical workflow but no learning curve effect for accuracy of implant positioning. Knee Surg Sports Traumatol Arthrosc 2019;27(4):1132–41.

29. Schopper C, Proier P, Luger M, et al. The learning curve in robotic assisted knee arthroplasty is flattened by the presence of a surgeon experienced with robotic assisted surgery. Knee Surg Sports Traumatol Arthrosc 2023;31(3):760.

The Medial Pivot Design in Total Knee Arthroplasty

Sydney M. Hodgeson, MD, Tatsuya Soeno, MD, Simon C. Mears, MD, PhD,
Jeffrey B. Stambough, MD, C. Lowry Barnes, MD, Benjamin M. Stronach, MS, MD*

KEYWORDS

- Total knee arthroplasty • Medial pivot • Adult reconstruction • Knee • Kinematics

KEY POINTS

- Medial pivot total knee arthroplasty implant designs function similar to that of the native knee with a relatively fixed medial center of rotation and a less conforming lateral compartment that follows an arcuate path.
- There are 2 types of TKA implants that attempt to reproduce the medial pivot pattern: those that were designed from the outset as medial pivot and those that are retrofitted to be medially congruent through a specifically designed polyethylene bearing.
- Existing literature on medial pivot implants have demonstrated high survivorship and patient outcomes compared to posterior stabilized implants.
- More studies are needed to compare newer medial pivot implants and retrofitted medial congruent implants due to the variations between implants.

INTRODUCTION

Total knee arthroplasty (TKA) has proven to be an effective surgical intervention for pain relief and functional improvement in patients with advanced knee osteoarthritis.[1] Despite this, approximately 20% of patients are not satisfied after TKA.[2] Instability is one of the 3 common reasons for revision, and there is a belief that underlying causes of pain could be from functional instability during activities of daily living loads.[3–5] Early TKA rationale focused on how to provide stability by retaining or sacrificing the cruciate ligaments, balancing flexion and extension gaps, and performing appropriate soft tissue balancing for varus and valgus knees. More recently, implant designs have attempted to provide improved stability through medial congruency, which more closely replicates native knee kinematics.[3,4] This review serves to provide readers with an overview of the rationale, characteristics, and outcomes relating to the class of medial pivot implants in TKA.

DISCUSSION

Rationale for Medial Pivot Design

For most of the twentieth century, knee kinematics were thought to function through the "four-bar link theory," which was first described by Zuppinger in 1904. According to this postulate, both the medial and lateral femoral condyles moved posteriorly in a uniform fashion under the control of the anterior and posterior cruciate ligaments.[5,6] However, the native knee was found to have asymmetric motion between the medial and lateral compartments, with more stability and less excursion through range of motion in the medial compartment than the lateral compartment (Fig. 1). Within the native medial compartment, there is increased conformity due to a larger medial femoral condyle, concave shape of the medial tibial plateau, and well-fixed medial meniscus in contrast to the smaller lateral femoral condyle and convex shape of the lateral tibial plateau. During normal native knee flexion, the lateral femoral condyle slides and rotates posteriorly on the tibial

Department of Orthopaedics, University of Arkansas for Medical Sciences, 4301 West Markham Street, Slot 531, Little Rock, AR 72205, USA
* Corresponding author.
E-mail address: BStronach@uams.edu

Orthop Clin N Am 55 (2024) 49–59
https://doi.org/10.1016/j.ocl.2023.06.007
0030-5898/24/

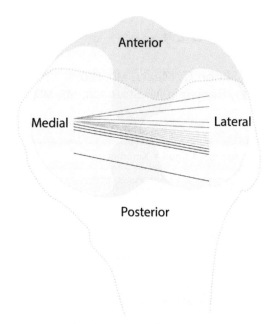

Fig. 1. Overhead projection of a native tibial plateau with the femur superimposed. The lines represent the contact point of the femur on the tibia in the medial and lateral compartments. The green lines represent extension to 30° of flexion, the yellow lines represent 30 to 90° of flexion and the red lines represent deep flexion.

plateau in an arcuate path while a more stable contact point is maintained between the medial femoral condyle and medial tibial plateau.[7] This results in a pivoting motion where the medial joint is fairly fixed and the lateral joint rotates about a medial center of rotation.[8]

Some cruciate retaining (CR) and posterior stabilizing (PS) TKA designs incorporate symmetric motion in the medial and lateral compartments, in contrast to that of the native knee.[8–10] When compared to native knees, both CR and PS designs have increased "paradoxic motion" with the femoral component sliding anteriorly on the tibial component during 30° to 60° knee flexion.[11–14] Although this can occur in both of these designs, more CR designs have been reported to have this paradoxic motion, possibly secondary to increased clinical and radiological laxity in CR designs and more consistent femoral rollback through the cam and post mechanism in PS designs.[12,15,16]

The medial pivot (MP) TKA was designed to recreate native knee motion as much as possible by using a spherical medial femoral condyle that articulates with a concave medial tibial plateau reinforced with an anterior lip (Fig. 2). This design increases the conformity of the medial compartment, referred to as a "ball-in-socket

articulation" that is similar in concept to the hip joint articulation. This creates a large contact area and decreases contact stress in the medial compartment, which prevents edge loading of the implant. The lateral femoral condyle of the medial pivot TKA moves freely on an arcuate path along the lateral tibial plateau with less conformity within the lateral compartment in an effort to simulate native knee kinematics.[12,16,17]

There are several different medial pivot TKA systems currently available on the market that were designed from inception to recreate medial pivot kinematic motion. With increasing popularity of the medial pivot TKA, several companies have developed medial pivot-like inserts to be retrofitted to function with their system's multi-radius femoral component to reproduce a more stable medial articulation. These new inserts are often described as "medial congruent," "medial stabilizing," or "medial dished" depending on the company jargon, and are ultimately designed to replicate the stability and possibly the kinematics of the MP TKAs while maintaining their original femoral and tibial components. One of the major differences between the 2 groups is whether the medial femoral condyle has a spherical single-radius (SR) curvature in both the anteroposterior and mediolateral planes or multi-radius (MR) of curvature in the sagittal plane. The spherical radius of curvature within the sagittal and coronal planes of the medial femoral condyle in TKAs originally designed as medial pivot produce a "ball-in-socket" articulation of the medial compartment of the knee. The SR TKA has a constant radius of curvature from 10° to 110° flexion to replicate the uniform flexion arc resulting from the isometric nature of the superficial medial collateral ligament throughout its range of motion.[18] Multi-radius (MR) femoral components, also referred to as a J curve, were designed with a larger radius of curvature anteriorly and a decreased radius posteriorly within the sagittal plane to increase flexion and femoral rollback.[19,20] MR implants have the characteristic of decreasing conformity with flexion, which may be an advantage for range of motion, but may potentially lead to flexion instability. Despite the theoretic advantages of SR, studies comparing single and multi-radius designs found no statistically significant differences in postoperative functional outcome, range of motion, or survival rate.[21–24]

PRIMARY MEDIAL PIVOT IMPLANT DESIGNS

Medial pivot TKA design varies with each manufacturer, and in recent years, inserts designed to

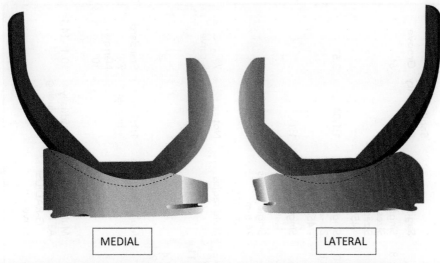

MEDIAL | LATERAL

Fig. 2. Sagittal cross-section of a medial pivot design TKA illustrating the increased conformity and anterior polyethylene height of the medial compartment in comparison to the lateral compartment.

increase medial conformity have become more readily available. There are two types of TKAs that attempt to reproduce the medial pivot pattern: those that were designed from the outset as medial pivot (MatOrtho, Medacta, Microport, Kyocera) and those that are retrofitted to be medially congruent through a specifically designed polyethylene bearing (Zimmer Biomet, Smith & Nephew, Johnson & Johnson). The details for both of these types of implants are provided in Tables 1–3.

Medacta GMK Sphere

The GMK Sphere was designed using information from the original medial pivot TKA, the FS1000. Medacta (Medacta International AG, Castel San Pietro, Switzerland) utilized an anthropometric database to determine implant sizing and fit. The GMK Sphere utilizes asymmetric femoral condyles (larger medial width than lateral width) to allow for increased surface contact area in the congruency of the medial femoral condyle and to shift the trochlea 2 mm lateral to midline for patellar tracking. The GMK Sphere femoral component is a cruciate retaining design. There are a total of 13 femoral component sizes (numbered 1–7 with + sizes for 1–6), each growing approximately 2 mm in the medial-lateral and anterior-posterior planes. There are two sphere sizes across the entire implant range with 25 mm sagittal radius of curvature for femoral sizes 1 to 3+ and 30 mm curvature for sizes 4 to 7. The tibial baseplate is asymmetric to match the native tibial geometry (2–4 mm larger anteroposterior medially than

laterally). There are 8 tibial implant sizes (size 1–6 and two transitional sizes at 3 and 4). The tibial polyethylene is manufactured to be the same congruency for sizes 1 to 3 tibial components (to match the 25 mm radius of the 1–3+ femurs) and for the 4 to 6 tibial components (to match the 30 mm radius of the 4–7 femurs). This allows for the mismatching of implant size within these two groups but requires transitional tibial baseplates to allow for a size 4 tibial tray to be used with the smaller sized femurs (1–3+) and a size 3 tibial tray to be used with the larger femurs (size 4–6). The femoral and tibial components are fabricated from cobalt chromium with cemented and press-fit options and a hypoallergenic titanium niobium nitride coated option. The ultra-high molecular weight tibial polyethylene comes in a standard formulation and a highly crosslinked vitamin E formulation with a sphere (MP) and cruciate retaining option available in both formulations.[25]

Microport Evolution

The Evolution (Microport, Memphis, TN) system is a second-generation implant based off the predecessor Advance (Wright Medical, Memphis, TN) Medial Pivot design. There is a cruciate retaining and a posterior stabilized option for femoral components with 8 femoral component sizes. The metal of the posterior femoral condyles is 1 to 2 mm thicker in comparison to the rest of the implant to provide greater contact area with the tibia in deep flexion. The sagittal radius of curvature varies based on femoral size from 21 mm to 29.9 mm and the system allows

Table 1
Technical specifications for femoral components of medial pivot designs

	Knee System	Sizes (n)	Overall A/P (mm)	Functional A/P (mm)	Overall M/L (mm)	Distal Condylar Thickness (mm)	Posterior Condylar Thickness (mm)	Sagittal Radius	Sagittal Conformity	Groove
Medial Pivot TKA	GMK® Sphere *Medacta*	13	53–77	38–58.5	56–80	Sizes 1–6+: 9 Size 7: 10	Sizes 1–6+: 8 Size 7: 9	*Single radius* Sizes 1–3: 25 mm Sizes 4–7: 30 mm –45°–115°	1:1	6°
	Evolution® MP knee *MicroPort*	8	47–65.5	30.5–48.3	55–73	9	Sizes 1–4: 10 Sizes 5–8: 11	*Single radius* 21–29.9 –45°–100°	1:1.04	3.6°
	SAIPH® *MatOrtho*	8	50–75	39–57	56–83	8–11	7–10	*Single radius*	1:1	-
	Physio-Knee® *KYOCERA*	5	56.3–67	40–50	58–74	8.5	9	*Single radius* 24 mm –45°–105°	1:1.01	5°
Retrofitted Medial Congruent/ Pivot TKA	Journey™ II CR/CS Medial Dished *Smith & Nephew*	10	51.7–79.8	Not measurable	59–82	*Medial* Sizes 1–8: 9.5 Sizes 9–10: 11.5 *Lateral* Sizes 1–8: 7 Sizes 9–10: 9	*Medial* Sizes 1–8: 9 Sizes 9–10: 11 *Lateral* Sizes 1–8: 7.4 Sizes 9–10: 9.4	*Multi radius*	Not constant	7° S-curve
	Persona® Medial Congruent *Zimmer Biomet*	21	48.1–75.2	41–65	55.5–77.5	9	9	*Multi radius*	1:1.1 or higher	Standard 7° Narrow 10°
	ATTUNE® CR Medial Stabilized *Johnson & Johnson*	14	47.7–76.1	46–73 (Sulcus AP)	54.1–82	9	8	*Multi radius* ATTUNE® G-RADIUS Curve	Gradually Reducing	10.1°–14.1°

Table 2
Inserts of individual medial pivot designs

	Knee System	Thickness (mm)	A/P (mm)	M/L (mm)	Articulating Geometry Shape	Lateral Arcuate Path	Anterior Medial Lip Height[a] (mm)	Posterior Medial Lip Height[a] (mm)
Medial Pivot TKA	GMK® Sphere Medacta	10–20	38–53	59–83	No slope	unconstrained	10	4
	Evolution® MP knee MicroPort	10–20	42–54	60–77	Bilateral: 3° posterior slope	15°	11 (CS) 10 (CR)	4.2 (CS) 2.0 (CR)
	SAIPH® MatOrtho	10–20	40–58	60–88	No slope	10°	11–14	5–7
	Physio-Knee® KYOCERA	8–16	38–48	62–78	Medial: Flat Lateral: 6° posterior slope	20°	9–11	1.5–2.2
Retrofitted Medial Congruent/Pivot TKA	Journey™ II CR Medial Dished Smith & Nephew	9–18	42–56	60–81	Medial: 5.5° posterior slope Lateral: 3.8° Posterior slope	Not publicly available	Not publicly available	Not publicly available
	Persona® Medial Congruent Zimmer Biomet	10–20	40.2–63.5	55.7–88.1	No slope	14°	10–13	3.1–3.4
	ATTUNE® CR Medial Stabilized Johnson & Johnson	9–20	39–54.2[b]	56–83[b]	No slope	along entire A-P length	9–11	2.3

[a] Definition of lip height may differ from each company.
[b] Entire size range is not commercially available at the time of preparing an article

Table 3
Tibial baseplates of individual medial pivot designs

	Knee System	Sizes (n)	Base Plate Posterior Slope
Medial Pivot TKA	GMK® Sphere *Medacta*	6	-
	Evolution® MP knee *MicroPort*	7	3°
	SAIPH® *MatOrtho*	6	7°
	Physio-Knee® *KYOCERA*	5	-
Retrofitted Medial Congruent/ Pivot TKA	Journey™ II CR Medial Dished *Smith & Nephew*	9	3°
	Persona® Medial Congruent *Zimmer Biomet*	9	5°
	ATTUNE® CR Medial Stabilized *Johnson & Johnson*	10	-

for one-up or one-down mismatch sizing between the femoral and tibial components. There are 7 tibial sizes that are asymmetric (larger anteroposterior medially than laterally) with 3° of posterior slope built into the stem and keel in relation to the baseplate. The tibial polyethylene has 3° of posterior slope laterally with a highly congruent (1:1.04) medial compartment with a 10 to 11 mm anterior lip and a 2.0 to 4.2 mm posterior lip. The lateral compartment is designed to allow for the femoral rotation of 15° in an arcuate path. There are three tibial polyethylene options to include cruciate substituting, cruciate retaining and posterior stabilized, all of which utilize the medial pivot design. The cruciate substituting design uses a cruciate retaining femur (does not require femoral box resection) but allows for excision of the PCL with the congruency of the tibial polyethylene providing stability. The femoral and tibial components are cobalt chromium with cemented and press-fit options and a hypoallergenic titanium niobium nitride coated option.

MatOrtho SAIPH

The SAIPH TKA is another second-generation medial pivot design that was preceded by the MatOrtho Medial Rotation Knee (MRK, MatOrtho, Surrey, UK). In this system, there are 8 femoral sizes (1–8) utilizing a spherical radius of curvature. The femoral component has asymmetric femoral condyles (larger medial width than lateral width) to shift the trochlea lateral to midline for patellar tracking. It is recommended to resect the anterior and posterior cruciate ligaments to allow the implant to function as designed with a cruciate substituting bearing used with a CR femoral implant design. There are 6 tibial implant sizes (size A-F) and some mismatching is permitted between femoral and tibial implant sizes (a guide is provided by MatOrtho to show compatibility). The tibial implant is a symmetric design (same anteroposterior dimension medially and laterally) and has 7° of posterior slope built into the stem and keel in relation to the baseplate. The baseplate has two anti-rotation pegs along with the stem and keel.

Kyocera Physio-Knee

The Physio-Knee system is a Medial Pivot TKA designed based on the bone morphology of Japanese people and has a medial single radius ball-and-socket design. The femoral component is a cruciate retaining design. There are 5 femoral component sizes, each growing approximately 4 mm in the medial-lateral and 2 to 3 mm anterior-posterior planes. The femoral component is made of high-purity alumina ceramic which has been reported to generate fewer polyethylene wear particles than metal femoral protheses.[26] The sagittal radius of curvature is the same for all femoral sizes (24 mm). The patellar groove is tilted 5° laterally to maintain high patellar conformity throughout knee range of motion. The tibial baseplate is asymmetric to match the native tibial geometry. There are 5 tibial implant sizes, and the sagittal radius of curvature is also the same for all sizes (24.3 mm). The system allows for one-up and one-down mismatch sizing between the femoral and tibial components. The anterior medial tibial polyethylene lip is 9–11 mm and posterior lip height is 15.-2.2 mm. The lateral side of the polyethylene has 6° posterior slope with 0° medial slope.

RETROFITTED MEDIAL CONGRUENT TOTAL KNEE ARTHROPLASTY SYSTEMS

Smith and Nephew Journey II Medial Dished

The Smith and Nephew Journey II Medial Dished system is a TKA system that was retrofitted from the Smith and Nephew Journey II cruciate retaining (CR) implant. In the Journey II system, there are 10 multi-radius femoral component sizes (1–10) with narrow implants available for female femoral morphology in sizes 3 to 6. The femoral components are cruciate retaining with asymmetric femoral condyles (increased medial distal and posterior condylar thickness) to mimic the biomechanics of the native knee. There are 9 tibial sizes that are asymmetric with 3° of posterior slope built into the stem in relation to the baseplate. Femoral and tibial sizing mismatch is tolerated in a variable range depending on the implant sizes with a chart available from the company providing these acceptable pairings. The tibial polyethylene has a constrained medial surface with a convex lateral surface to allow for femoral rollback. Due to this, the polyethylene thickness centrally is 2.5 mm thicker in the lateral compartment compared to the medial compartment and there is a greater differential in the medial compartment between the central thickness and anterior lip height (6–10 mm) as compared to the lateral compartment (4–7 mm).

Zimmer Biomet Persona Medial Congruent

The Zimmer Biomet Persona (Warsaw, IN) system was initially designed with CR, ultracongruent and PS bearing options and later added a medial congruent bearing option. There are 12 femoral implant sizes with narrow options available in sizes 3 to 11. The tibial baseplates were designed using a bone morphology database to better match the spectrum of anatomic sizes. There are 9 tibial implant sizes. The baseplates are asymmetric with a larger medial anteroposterior width than lateral and the implant sizes grow in a disproportionate manner. The medial congruent bearing is intended for use with the CR femur. The allowable sizing mismatch for the femur to the tibial polyethylene is narrower than the other bearing offerings (ultracongruent, CR, PS) due to the increased conformity and resultant need for closer size matching. A chart

is provided and should be referenced for surgeons accustomed to using the other bearing options. The tibial polyethylene has a medial anterior lip height of 10 to 13 mm which allows for minimal anteroposterior translation (~3 mm) within the medial compartment while reduced conformity in the lateral compartment allows for ~11 mm of anteroposterior translation. The PCL can be resected or retained by the surgeon based on surgeon preference and intra-operative findings.

Depuy Attune Medial Stabilized

The Depuy Attune (Warsaw, IN, USA) system was initially designed to utilize a congruent or posterior stabilized bearing and later added a medial stabilized bearing. The system utilizes a femoral component with a gradually reducing radius of curvature design (termed GRADIUS) based on the J-curve concept. It is size-specific based on anthropomorphic variations that were determined utilizing an anatomic database to optimize radius of curvature and ideal fit based on femoral size.[27] There are ten femoral sizes with narrow options available in sizes 3 to 6. The Attune (Warsaw, IN, USA) system has CR and PS femurs along with fixed bearing and rotating platform options but the medial stabilized bearing is designed for use with the CR femur and fixed bearing tibia. There are 10 tibial baseplate sizes. The tibial baseplate utilizes a central locking mechanism termed LogicLock that does not require a peripheral locking rim. This allows for a 2 up/2 down sizing mismatch between the femur and tibial baseplate. The system is designed so the tibial polyethylene matches the femoral implant size and not the tibial baseplate size. This provides maximal conformity between the femoral profile and the tibial polyethylene. The medial stabilized polyethylene is designed to have a congruent medial compartment for minimal anteroposterior translation. The lateral compartment is flat in the central section to allow for rollback in mid-flexion with slight anterior and posterior concave curvature that is designed to limit excessive translation but allow for anteroposterior motion.

OUTCOMES
Kinematics and Function

The kinematics and function of the medial pivot (MP) TKA, specifically Microport Evolution, Microport Advance, Medacta GMK sphere, MatOrtho MRK and MatOrtho SAIPH, have been studied. Kato, and colleagues, recently published a prospective study comparing the translational stability and outcomes of 71

Evolution medial pivot TKAs with 51 DePuy Attune posterior-stabilizing (PS) implants. They measured the anterior translation of the tibia relative to the femur at 30° and 60° of knee flexion with an arthrometer at 6 months postoperatively. They found that patients in the Microport Evolution MP TKA group had significantly decreased the anterior translation of the tibia relative to the femur compared to the Attune PS group at 60° flexion and no significant difference in anterior translation at 30° knee flexion, suggesting increased anterior-posterior stability with increasing knee flexion. Moreover, there was no difference in post-operative ROM at 6 months and 1-year between groups.[28] Barnes and colleagues conducted a radiographic study comparing 9 Microport Advance MP TKAs and cruciate-retaining Advance Double-High TKAs using fluoroscopy while standing, mid-kneeling, and kneeling. They found that the anterior lip of the MP implant prevented anterior "paradoxic" motion of the femur during flexion, indicating that kneeling would be safe with MP TKAs.[17] Scott, and colleagues performed static and dynamic assessments in weightbearing and non-weightbearing activities using pulsed fluoroscopy in 15 patients with Medacta GMK Sphere implants. They found the GMK sphere medial pivot TKA functions as intended with kinematics similar to the native knee with a fixed medial point of rotation and lateral excursion.[29] A similar study involving the fluoroscopic evaluation of 4 activities to include stepping up and down, lunges, kneeling, and pivoting was performed with 14 patients with MatOrtho SAIPH TKA implants. The knees demonstrated the asymmetric posterior translation of the lateral femur in flexion with a fixed medial point of rotation without anterior "paradoxic" motion of the femur during active weight-bearing and deep knee flexion in a similar manner to the native knee. Additionally, patients in this study had a mean maximal knee flexion of 127° (100°-155°).[30] Hossain, and colleagues performed a prospective study comparing ROM of 40 patients with the DePuy Press Fit Condylar Sigma posterior stabilizing (PS) knee with 42 patients with the MatOrtho MRK. In their study, patients with the MRK implant had higher overall knee ROM at 1 year post-operatively with the medial pivot knee (114.9°) compared to patients with PS knees (100.1°).[31]

Patient Satisfaction

There have been multiple studies assessing patient satisfaction with medial pivot implants, with most focusing on the Microport Advance

design and more recently the Microport Evolution. Kato and colleagues recently published a study demonstrating that patients with the Microport Evolution MP TKA design had significantly improved visual analogue scale (VAS) for pain, 2011 Knee Society Score (KSS), and Forgotten Joint Score (FSS) compared to the Attune PS TKA. Interestingly, there was a negative correlation between anterior translation distance and the KSS function score, suggesting that the MP TKA may contribute to improved postoperative function compared to PS TKAs.[28] Schmidt and colleagues assessed the clinical and radiographic results of 373 patients receiving the Microport Advance medial pivot TKA and found patients had a higher average postoperative Knee Society Score (KSS) of 95.5 with approximately 98% of patients having excellent or good results.[32] Bianchi, and colleagues performed a retrospective cohort study comparing the function and outcomes of 16 patients with Microport Evolution medial pivot TKA implants with 16 Zimmer Biomet Persona posterior-stabilizing (PS) TKAs. They found that patients with the Microport Evolution medial pivot TKAs had significantly higher postoperative Forgotten Joint Scores in comparison to the PS group.[33] Batra, and colleagues performed a study with 53 patients who received simultaneous bilateral TKAs with the Microport Advance medial pivot implant in one knee and the Smith and Nephew Genesis II PS implant in the other knee. They found patients had better Knee Society Scores (KSS) in the MP knee compared to the contralateral PS knee at 3 months, 6 months, and 4 years post-operatively.[34] However, in another study by Lin, and colleagues comparing 121 patients with the Microport Advance MP TKA and 332 patients with PS TKAs (219 Zimmer NexGen, 113 Stryker Scorpio), they found no difference in pain or satisfaction according to Numeric Rating Scale pain score and five-level satisfaction ratings, respectively.[35] Regarding the MatOrtho MRKknee, Hossain, and colleagues found that patients had improved Western Ontario and McMaster Universities Osteoarthritis Index (WOMAC) pain subscores and the physical component of the 36-Item Short Form Survey (SF-36) compared to patients with DePuy Press-Fit Condylar Sigma posterior stabilizing (PS) TKAs.[31]

Survivorship

There is currently limited survivorship data available on MP TKAs as fewer of these knees have been implanted in comparison to other systems, but the currently available data is consistent with non-inferior survivorship. Alessio-Mazzola et. al. conducted a systematic review of 34 studies that included a total of 3377 medial pivot TKAs with an overall high survivorship with a 1.9% revision rate after 10 years.[36] Cassar-Gheiti, et. al., conducted a meta-analysis in 2020 to study the survivorship of medial-pivot knees analyzing 25 studies and 5 different registries to include the National Joint Registry, Australian Orthopedic Association National Joint Registry, Dutch Arthroplasty Register, the New Zealand Orthopedic Association Joint Registry, and the Michigan Arthroplasty Collaborative Quality Initiative. The implants included in the meta-analysis included Microport Advance MP, MatOrtho MRK, Alumina Medial Pivot, MatOrtho SAIPH, Zimmer Biomet Persona MC, and Microport Evolution Medial Pivot. They found that the mean survivorship free of aseptic loosening for the medial pivot TKAs was 99% at 6.9 years.[37] Øhrn and colleagues, conducted a study on the survivorship and cause for revision for medial pivot TKAs using data from the Norwegian Arthroplasty Register and the Australian Orthopedic Association National Joint Registry. The medial pivot implants from the Australian registry included the Microport Evolution, the MatOrtho MRK, the MatOrtho SAIPH, the GMK Sphere, and the Microport Advance while the Norwegian registry only included the Microport Advance II, the Microport Evolution, and the GMK sphere. Within the Australian registry, 9% of all TKAs were medial pivot knees, and there was an increased revision risk with the Microport Advance and the GMK sphere medial pivot implants compared to PS knees with infection being the most common cause for revision (27%). Within the Norwegian registry, 1% of all TKAs were medial pivot knees, and there was no difference in revision risk between the medial pivot knees and PS knees with loosening and instability being the most common cause of revision.[38] Karachalios and colleagues and Macheras and colleagues conducted studies assessing the long-term survivorship of the Microport Advance MP knee with similar survivorship of 97.3% at 15 years and 98.8% at 17 years, respectively between the two studies.[39,40]

There is currently a lack of literature available regarding the function, patient satisfaction and survivorship of retrofitted medial congruent bearing designs as these bearings have been on the market for a short period of time. There are differences amongst these retrofitted bearings, and differences when compared to MP TKA designs. The effects of these differences regarding outcomes is currently unknown. The increasing popularity of these designs will provide an increasing cohort of patients that can be studied regarding the long-term outcomes of these designs.

SUMMARY

In conclusion, the medial pivot TKA design functions similar to that of the native knee with a fixed medial center of rotation and a less conforming lateral compartment that follows an arcuate path. The medial pivot TKA has seen increasing popularity with more companies offering medial pivot or medial congruent bearings. It is important to note that there are variations in the design features and rationale between these different MP implant offerings. According to the existing literature, most medial pivot designs had overall high survivorship and improved or similar range of motion when compared to PS designs. Although improved patient satisfaction with medial pivot TKAs has been demonstrated, these studies involve different implants with their own design variations. Further studies are needed to compare the outcomes and survivorship of more recent medial pivot TKAs with each other.

CLINICS CARE POINTS

- Medial pivot design TKA utilizes a highly congruent medial bearing and less conforming lateral bearing to reproduce native knee kinematics.

- The medial pivot TKA is amenable to press fit or cemented surgical technique.

- The use of medial pivot TKA for primary TKA is increasing in popularity while longer term data is required to determine the potential benefits of this design when compared to traditional bearing types.

ACKNOWLEDGMENTS

The authors would like to recognize the contribution of Alexa Pearce for designing and drawing the included illustrations and for assistance with editing and generation of the article.

REFERENCES

1. Choi YJ, Ra HJ. Patient satisfaction after total knee arthroplasty. Knee Surg Relat Res 2016;28(1):1–15.

2. Tolk J, van der Steen M, Janssen R, et al. Total Knee Arthroplasty: What to Expect? A Survey of the Members of the Dutch Knee Society on Long-Term Recovery after Total Knee Arthroplasty. J Knee Surg 2017;30(06):612–6.

3. Bosch LC, Beger SB, Duncan ST, et al. Intraoperative Practice Variability in Total Knee Arthroplasty. J Arthroplasty 2020;35(3):725–31.

4. Schmidt R, Komistek RD, Blaha JD, et al. Fluoroscopic analyses of cruciate-retaining and Medial Pivot knee implants. Clin Orthop Relat Res 2003; 410:139–47. Lippincott Williams and Wilkins.

5. Rong GW, Wang YC. The role of cruciate ligaments in maintaining knee joint stability. Clin Orthop Relat Res 1987;215:65–71.

6. Zuppinger H. Die aktive Flexion im unbelasteten Kniegelenk. Zuricher Habil Schr, Wisebaden: Bergmann. Published online 1904;703–63.

7. Komistek RD, Dennis DA, Mahfouz M. In vivo fluoroscopic analysis of the normal human knee. Clin Orthop Relat Res 2003;410:69–81. Lippincott Williams and Wilkins.

8. Sabatini L, Risitano S, Parisi G, et al. Medial pivot in total knee arthroplasty: Literature review and our first experience. Clin Med Insights Arthritis Musculoskelet Disord 2018;11. https://doi.org/10.1177/1179544117751431.

9. Moewis P, Hommel H, Trepczynski A, et al. Weight Bearing Activities change the Pivot Position after Total Knee Arthroplasty. Sci Rep 2019;9(1). https://doi.org/10.1038/s41598-019-45694-y.

10. Becher C, Heyse TJ, Kron N, et al. Posterior stabilized TKA reduce patellofemoral contact pressure compared with cruciate retaining TKA in vitro. Knee Surg Sports Traumatol Arthrosc 2009;17(10): 1159–65.

11. Dennis DA, Komistek RD, Colwell CE, et al. In Vivo Anteroposterior Femorotibial Translation of Total Knee Arthroplasty: A Multicenter Analysis. Clin Orthop Relat Res 1998;356:47–57. Lippincott Williams & Wilkins. http://journals.lww.com/clinorthop.

12. Blaha JD. A medial pivot geometry. Orthopedics 2002;25(9):963–4.

13. Putame G, Terzini M, Rivera F, et al. Kinematics and kinetics comparison of ultra-congruent versus medial-pivot designs for total knee arthroplasty by multibody analysis. Sci Rep 2022;12(1). https://doi.org/10.1038/s41598-022-06909-x.

14. Dejour D, Deschamps G, Garotta L, et al. Laxity in posterior cruciate sparing and posterior stabilized total knee prostheses. Clin Orthop Relat Res 1999;364:182–93.

15. Victor J, Banks S, Bellemans J, et al. Bellemans " J. Kinematics of posterior cruciate ligament-retaining and-substituting total knee arthroplasty A prospective randomised outcome study. J Bone Joint Surg 2005. https://doi.org/10.1302/0301-620X.87B5.

16. Barnes CL, Blaha JD, DeBoer D, et al. Assessment of a Medial Pivot Total Knee Arthroplasty Design in a Cadaveric Knee Extension Test Model. J Arthroplasty 2012;27(8). https://doi.org/10.1016/j.arth.2012.02.008.

17. Barnes CL, Sharma A, Blaha JD, et al. Kneeling Is Safe for Patients Implanted With Medial-Pivot Total Knee Arthroplasty Designs. J Arthroplasty 2011; 26(4):549–54.

18. Shimizu N, Tomita T, Yamazaki T, et al. In vivo movement of femoral flexion axis of a single-radius total knee arthroplasty. J Arthroplasty 2014; 29(12):2407–11.

19. Iwaki H, Pinskerova V, Freeman MAR. Tibiofemoral movement 1: The shape and relative movements of the femur and tibia in the unloaded cadaver knee. Journal of Bone and Joint Surgery - Series B 2000; 82(8):1189–95.

20. Ng JWG, Bloch BV, James PJ. Sagittal radius of curvature, trochlea design and ultracongruent insert in total knee arthroplasty. EFORT Open Rev 2019;4(8):519–24.

21. Jo AR, Song EK, Lee KB, et al. A comparison of stability and clinical outcomes in single-radius versus multi-radius femoral design for total knee arthroplasty. J Arthroplasty 2014;29(12):2402–6.

22. Liu S, Long H, Zhang Y, et al. Meta-Analysis of Outcomes of a Single-Radius Versus Multi-Radius Femoral Design in Total Knee Arthroplasty. J Arthroplasty 2016;31(3):646–54.

23. Kim J, Min KD, Lee BI, et al. Comparison of functional outcomes between single-radius and multi-radius femoral components in primary total knee arthroplasty: a meta-analysis of randomized controlled trials. Knee Surg Relat Res 2020;32(1). https://doi.org/10.1186/S43019-020-00067-Y.

24. Indelli PF, Morello F, Ghirardelli S, et al. No clinical differences at the 2-year follow-up between single radius and J-curve medial pivot total knee arthroplasty in the treatment of neutral or varus knees. Knee Surg Sports Traumatol Arthrosc 2020;28(12):3949–54.

25. Medacta International. GMK Sphere. Specification Guide. 2020; https://media.medacta.com/media/gmk-sphere-specification-guide-9926sphere11sgus-rev01.pdf.

26. Minoda Y, Kobayashi A, Iwaki H, et al. Polyethylene wear particle generation in vivo in an alumina medial pivot total knee prosthesis. Biomaterials 2005;26(30):6034–40.

27. Depuy Synthes. Attune® Knee System. https://www.jnjmedtech.com/en-US/product/attune-medial-stabilized-knee-system.

28. Kato M, Warashina H, Mitamura S, et al. Medial pivot-based total knee arthroplasty achieves better clinical outcomes than posterior-stabilised total knee arthroplasty. Knee Surg Sports Traumatol Arthrosc 2022. https://doi.org/10.1007/s00167-022-07149-2.

29. Scott G, Imam MA, Eifert A, et al. Can a total knee arthroplasty be both rotationally unconstrained and anteroposteriorly stabilised? A pulsed fluoroscopic investigation. Bone Joint Res 2016;5(3): 80–6.

30. Shimmin A, Martinez-Martos S, Owens J, Iorgulescu AD, Banks S. Fluoroscopic Motion Study Confirming the Stability of a Medial Pivot Design Total Knee Arthroplasty. Knee 2015;22:522–6.

31. Hossain F, Patel S, Rhee SJ, et al. Knee arthroplasty with a medially conforming ball-and-socket tibiofemoral articulation provides better function. Clin Orthop Relat Res 2011;469:55–63. Springer New York LLC.

32. Schmidt R, Ogden S, Blaha JD, et al. Midterm clinical and radiographic results of the medial pivot total knee system. Int Orthop 2014;38(12):2495–8.

33. Bianchi N, Facchini A, Mondanelli N, et al. Medial pivot vs posterior stabilized total knee arthroplasty designs: A gait analysis study. Med Glas 2021;18(1): 1–8.

34. Batra S, Malhotra R, Kumar V, et al. Superior patient satisfaction in medial pivot as compared to posterior stabilized total knee arthroplasty: a prospective randomized study. Knee Surg Sports Traumatol Arthrosc 2021;29(11):3633–40.

35. Lin Y, Chen X, Li L, et al. Comparison of Patient Satisfaction Between Medial Pivot Prostheses and Posterior-Stabilized Prostheses in Total Knee Arthroplasty. Orthop Surg 2020;12(3):836–42.

36. Alessio-Mazzola M, Clemente A, Russo A, et al. Clinical radiographic outcomes and survivorship of medial pivot design total knee arthroplasty: a systematic review of the literature. Arch Orthop Trauma Surg 2022. https://doi.org/10.1007/s00402-021-04210-6.

37. Cassar-Gheiti AJ, Jamieson PS, Radi M, et al. Evaluation of the Medial Stabilized Knee Design Using Data From National Joint Registries and Current Literature. J Arthroplasty 2020;35(7):1950–5.

38. Øhrn FD, Gøthesen Ø, Låstad Lygre SH, et al. Decreased Survival of Medial Pivot Designs Compared with Cruciate-retaining Designs in TKA Without Patellar Resurfacing. Clin Orthop Relat Res 2020;478(6):1207–18.

39. Karachalios T, Varitimidis S, Bargiotas K, et al. An 11- to 15-year clinical outcome study of the Advance Medial Pivot total knee arthroplasty: Pivot knee arthroplasty. Bone and Joint Journal 2016;98-B(8):1050–5.

40. Macheras GA. A Long Term Clinical Outcome of the Medial Pivot Knee Arthroplasty System. Knee 2017;24.

Intraoperative Medial Instability During Total Knee Arthroplasty

Zachary Aberman, MD[a,1], James Germano, MD[b,2],
Giles R. Scuderi, MD[c,3,*]

KEYWORDS

- MCL • Intraoperative • Injury • Total knee replacement • Repair • Outcomes

KEY POINTS

- The incidence of intraoperative medial collateral ligament (MCL) injury is likely under-reported and there is a paucity of research on the subject.
- There are pre-operative risk factors that increase the likelihood of having a MCL injury during total knee arthroplasty (TKA).
- Care must be taken during the approach and surgical steps of TKA to prevent inadvertent injury to the MCL.
- MCL injury must be fully assessed when it does happen, and a plan to manage should be undertaken with a focus on obtaining a balanced knee through the range of motion.
- Missed MCL injury or postoperative medial laxity can lead to an increased rate of revision and TKA complication.

INTRODUCTION

Total knee arthroplasty (TKA) is a successful and increasingly commonly performed procedure in the United States. Growth models project up to almost 1 million procedures annually by the year 2030 with an American pool of potential operative candidates growing up to 3 million people by that time.[1] There are several techniques and alignment goals employed during TKA and there is conflicting data as the best approach. However, a common denominator to all these approaches is stability, and the profound importance that maintaining stability through the range of motion has on a successful TKA outcome.

The medial collateral ligament (MCL) is the major supporting structure during valgus and rotatory stress. Injury and/or laxity to the static and dynamic medial stabilizers of the knee after TKA can have a significant impact on the balance and stability of the TKA throughout the range of motion. Prevention and timely identification of medial instability when it does occur is critical to having a successful outcome. The incidence of medial instability during TKA is hard to quantify; studies have shown rates from 0.43% to 3%.[2] However, the incidence is likely underreported and is managed at the time of surgery without additional notation or documentation.[2] These medial instability events have been shown, even when properly managed, to lead to a concomitant increase in revision rates.[2]

Risk factors to medial instability can be multifactorial including both anatomic and surgical. Preoperative evaluation should identify the

[a] Lenox Hill Hospital Northwell Health, NY, USA; [b] Long Island Valley Stream Hospital Northwell Health, Valley Stream, NY, USA; [c] Department of Orthopaedic Surgery, Lenox Hill, New York, NY, USA
[1] Present address: 11 Black Hall 130 East 77th Street, New York, NY 10075, USA
[2] Present address: 444 Merrick Road, Lynbrook, NY 11563, USA
[3] Present Address: 210 East 64th Street, New York, NY 10065, USA
* Corresponding author. 1001 Franklin Avenue, Suite 110, Garden City, NY 11530
E-mail address: gscuderi@northwell.edu

Orthop Clin N Am 55 (2024) 61–71
https://doi.org/10.1016/j.ocl.2023.06.005

degree of deformity, integrity of the MCL, and anatomic considerations, which may influence the surgical plan and implant choice.[3,4] Iatrogenic injury to the MCL may also occur during the surgical approach, bone preparation, soft tissue release for a fixed varus deformity, or accidental transection.[5–7]

Management of intraoperative medial instability during TKA can be addressed in several different ways depending on the nature of the injury and the type of implant system. The options include, but are not limited to, primary repair, repair and augmentation with autograft/allograft or synthetic product, fixation with screws and washer constructs, increasing polyethylene thickness, or increasing prosthetic constraint.[4,8–14] Each of these options has advantages and disadvantages and depends on the type of injury and degree of instability.

ANATOMIC CONSIDERATIONS

The medial soft tissue supporting structures, which contribute to the stability of the knee, are composed of both dynamic and static stabilizers. The static stabilizers include the extra-articular ligamentous structures, the deep and superficial medial collateral ligaments, the posterior oblique collateral ligament (POL), and the joint capsule. Dynamic stabilizers to the medial knee include multiple muscular structures. The semimembranosus tenses the posteromedial capsule of the knee at its attachment just proximal to the superficial MCL on the tibia. Its tension changes throughout active range of motion of the knee both passively and actively contributing to medial stability. The medial retinaculum, as an extension of the vastus medialis aponeurosis, can dynamically stabilize the knee as well. As the vastus medialis contracts the distal fibers of the aponeurosis, which are affixed to the anterior portions of the medial capsule, are tightened and the anteromedial knee is stabilized while the knee extends from the pull of the quadriceps.[15]

The MCL is divided into deep and superficial ligaments. The superficial MCL is the largest structure over the medial knee with 1 femoral attachment and 2 tibial attachments. It inserts proximal and posterior to the medial epicondyle of the femur then courses distally to the tibia. The first attachment is to the soft tissue envelope over the anterior arm of the semimembranousus, which is attached to the tibia.[16] The inferior medial geniculate artery and vein runs between the tibia and the superficial MCL at this level. At its second insertion more distal,

the superficial MCL has a broad-based attachment just anterior to the posteromedial crest of the tibia forming the floor of the pes anserine bursa approximately 6 cm distal to the joint line.[16,17]

The deep MCL structure is fundamentally a thickening of the medial capsule of the knee with a distinct density at the anterior border where it runs parallel to the superficial MCL. Posteriorly the deep MCL blends into the central arm of the POL. Proximally and distally the deep MCL directly connects to the femur and tibia through a soft tissue confluence with meniscofemoral and meniscotibial attachments. The meniscotibial connection, of the deep MCL, inserts directly on the medial tibial plateau at edge of the articular cartilage. The attachment continues distally below the joint line where it is also intimately intertwined with the capsule and the medial meniscus. The superficial MCL lies directly superficial to this structure at this level. This exposes the deep and superficial MCL fibers to potential injury during the resection of medial meniscus and any medial tibial bone resection during TKA.

The POL connects the semimembranosus tendon to the femur as well as attaching to the tibia and the capsule of the posteromedial knee. The POL merges with the posterior fibers of the superficial MCL and is primarily at risk during resection of the posterior medial portion of the medial meniscus and saw cuts to the posteromedial corner of the tibia.[16]

ETIOLOGY OF INJURY, RISK FACTORS, AND PREVENTION

Injury to the medial structures can occur at any time during surgery. Meticulous surgical technique should be undertaken during surgical dissection, soft tissue release, and bone resection. Care should be taken during exposure of a stiff knee, forceful manipulation of the knee, or during retractor placement and retraction, may cause injury or avulsion of the MCL. Tibial avulsions of the MCL most commonly occur during hyperflexion for exposure of the knee[9] but can also occur from the femoral attachment on osteoporotic bone. The MCL is also susceptible to direct injury from the excursion of the saw blade during bone resection of the tibia and femur.[3,7]

Both modifiable and nonmodifiable factors can increase the risk of damaging the medial structures during TKA including preoperative limb alignment, joint contractures, and patient habitus. Patients with preoperative tibiofemoral alignment in severe varus (>7°), medial instability with a valgus deformity, morbid obesity, and preoperative flexion contracture have been reported as a risk of MCL injury.[4,18,19] A cup and saucer morphology where the distal femur is articulating over a proximal tibial bone defect leads to a relative increased slope has also been described as an independent risk factor.[20]

There are several intraoperative factors that also need to be understood. Use of larger oscillating saw blades, which are wider than the femoral condyle, has been shown to be a risk factor for MCL injury.[3] In correcting a fixed varus deformity, the appropriate sequence of steps in soft tissue release should include osteophyte removal followed by medial soft tissue release. The late removal of osteophytes has also been implicated in creating too much medial laxity during TKA.[3] Extensive early soft-tissue releases, overly strenuous testing of varus valgus stability of the knee with trials in place, aggressive hyperflexion or forced subluxation of the tibia with trials in place for visualization, abrupt forceful retraction, and placing overly tight trials in while in flexion are all controllable risk factors for causing medial injury.[3–6,18,19]

As we can see from this long list, there are many potential ways to injure the medial stabilizing structures of the knee during the procedure. The key to minimizing any unintentional injury to these structures requires taking a consistent stepwise approach to performing TKA, having knowledge of the above-described anatomy, and taking an active role to protect them throughout the procedure.

The approach to the knee during a standard medial parapatellar approach to the knee involves elevating the retinaculum and capsular attachments to the medial proximal tibial plateau. A careful evaluation of the preoperative ligamentous balance of the knee is paramount to completing any approach to the knee in such a way as to not excessively release any medial tissues from the tibia which will affect the future balance of the TKA. A general rule of thumb is to start with a minimal release of the medial soft tissues and to remain at the level of the parameniscal soft tissue and the joint line.[3] Release along the joint line to the level of the mid-coronal plane will preserve the more posterior, capsular, deep MCL, and POL attachments to the tibia. Stopping at the mid-coronal plane has been advocated in patients with neutral or minimal varus deformity to prevent overreleasing these structures prematurely and affecting the ultimate balance.[12] In a more severe varus

deformity and knees with significant medial soft tissue contracture this joint line release may be taken around the posteromedial corner with subperiosteal elevation, sharp dissection, or electrocautery. Care must be taken to stay on bone when releasing around the posteromedial corner and it is possible to encounter the inferomedial geniculate vessel at this level when deep to the superficial MCL[16] (Fig. 1).

The release of the medial capsule during the initial approach may be accomplished by sharp dissection or electrocautery with care taken to maintain integrity of the soft-tissue envelope and to always remain on bone during subperiosteal elevation. Transverse disruption of distal periosteum can lead to difficulties with later closer of the arthrotomy. This can affect medial stability as well as preventing watertight closure of the arthrotomy.

Minimally invasive surgical techniques including subvastus and midvastus approaches have limited evidence of increasing the risk of MCL injury during TKA[21–23] Regardless of the approach taken to perform the TKA, the location and careful placement of retractors is paramount to protecting the medial knee. Retractors placed on the medial side of the knee during TKA serve 2 primary goals. The first goal of retractors is to improve the visualization of the necessary anatomy to complete the surgery. The second goal is to protect structures from unintentional injury. There are many different retractors to choose from on the market and they come in various shapes and sizes, with both blunt and sharp tips.

During subperiosteal dissection of the medial capsule it is important to keep the tissues retracted medially to allow the surgeon to visualize the soft tissue to bone interface; this can be accomplished with various types of retractors

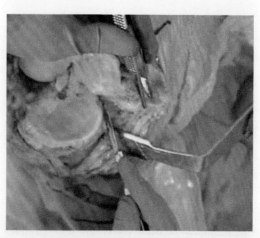

Fig. 1. Posteromedial release of soft tissue off of tibia.

Without appropriate visualization it is possible to inadvertently skive into the soft tissue envelope, which could lead to transection of the capsule or other deeper structures as described above.

The position of deeper medial retractors may change depending on the patient's anatomy and existing soft tissue balance/alignment.

Medial Retraction During Tibial Preparation

Medial retraction during tibial preparation should be designed to protect the skin, retinaculum, deep and superficial MCL. When there is a fixed varus deformity and a medial soft tissue release is performed from the proximal tibia, the tip of the retractor can be seated on the proximal tibial bone extending around the posteromedial joint line. A retractor is placed horizontally deep enough to stop the saw blade excursion into the soft tissues at the level of the planned tibial resection (Fig. 2). In the case of a valgus deformity, it is important that the MCL is protected during tibial resection. Although the placement of these retractors is crucial for protection, they are also a potential source of injury, as this location is just deep to the remaining intact deep MCL and superficial MCL fibers. If the medial retractor is pulled too hard to obtain visualization it is possible to cause an avulsion to the distal attachment of the deep and superficial MCL footprints described above. Surgeons using mobile window incisions, mini-incisions, or with certain robotic platforms may alternate between placing lateral tibial and medial tibial retractors during resection of the tibia. Additional superficial soft tissue retractors or self-retainers may also be used during the tibia resection to prevent damage to those tissues by saw blade oscillation. Retraction and protection of the lateral structures and the patella tendon are also key to a successful tibial

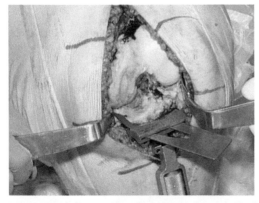

Fig. 2. Medial retractor placement prior to tibial resection.

resection. A detail orientated approach to protecting these structures is paramount, but outside the scope of this current review.

Medial Retraction During Femoral Preparation

The medial soft tissue also needs to be protected during preparation of the femur including during osteophyte resection and bone resection. The retractor is placed deep to the deep MCL at the level of the joint line. This will retract the deep MCL, the superficial MCL, and the capsule as these structures insert more posteriorly behind the medial epicondyle. It is important that all these structures are retracted adequately to visualize the soft tissue insertions and remove osteophytes. During the resection of medial femoral osteophytes, it is important to carefully dissect them off from any soft-tissue attachments to avoid unintended injury to the MCL.

Once the resection guide is in place or the robotic saw is ready for femoral resections, the medial retractor should be double checked to ensure it is deep to the deep MCL. The position of this retractor should be reassessed throughout femoral resection. It may become necessary to change the angle of the retractor when transitioning from distal femur, posterior femur, and posterior chamfer cuts to have the retractor in line with the saw blades excursion path and maintain protection. The MCL appears to be at the highest risk during the resection of the posterior femoral condyle.[9]

MANAGEMENT OF MEDIAL INSTABILITY

Once a discrete injury or medial ligamentous instability is identified during a TKA, there are several options for how to address the issue. In the setting of a sharp transection of the MCL whether caused by an errant saw blade, knife, or electrocautery, the first step is a careful evaluation of the extent of the injury, if operating through a minimally invasive approach it may be necessary to extend the incision to fully visualize the injury. Once the injury is fully assessed a decision needs to be made as to the extent of the injury and the method of managing it.

Authors have advocated a myriad of techniques for addressing unanticipated medial instability during TKA.[4,8–14] In the setting of mid-substance MCL injury, usually the fibers of the MCL are disrupted and a direct end-to-end repair has been suggested. Several studies show that primary repair of a sharp dissection can be achieved without negatively affecting the balancing of the TKA.[8,10] However, this finding may be difficult to generalize to all surgeries as the majority of patients in these cohorts used cruciate retaining (CR) components with preservation of the PCL, which contributes to medial stability. Several authors describe the importance of completing any remaining bony preparation of the knee prior to repairing the injury.[8,12] This is important as overtightening of the MCL during the repair procedure could detrimentally affect the balance of the medial side of the TKA. After the preparation is completed for the TKA, the knee is brought into extension and a spacer block equal to the size of the completed construct is inserted or the trials are retained. The repair of the ends of the torn ligament is brought together with either a Krakow, Kessler, or barrel stitching style technique using nonabsorbable high strength suture (Fig. 3). The goal is to tension the soft tissues to the space created by the spacer block or trial. When the injury is not complete, this technique has also been applied, with repair of the injured fibers being accomplished in a similar manner with the spacer block or knee construct in place with the knee between 30° of flexion and full extension. It has also been advocated to evaluate the injury before the end of the case and wait to complete the full repair until after final components are in. This will help prevent damage to the repair during final implantation of TKA components.

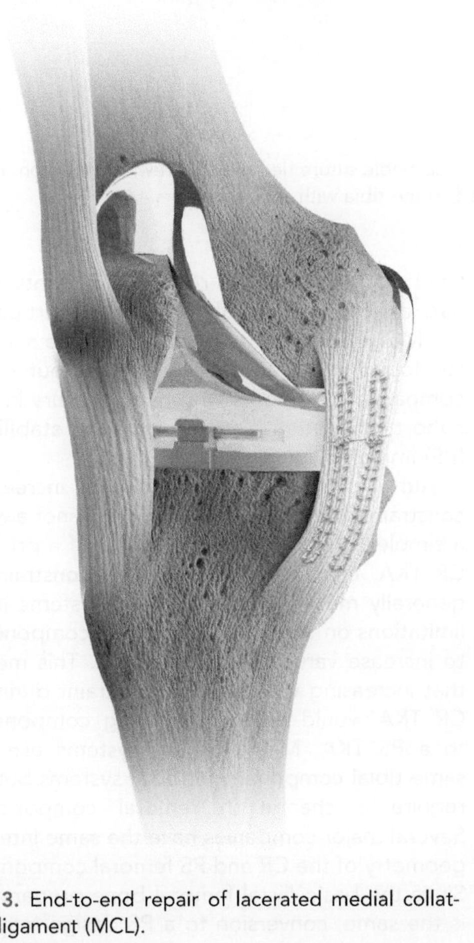

When the injured MCL is not able to be approximated end to end authors advocate for several other potential options. One option is to augment the repair with a woven high strength nonabsorbable commercial product, autograft, or a cadaver allograft tissue[8,12,24] (Fig. 4). This technique also requires careful tensioning of the repair with regard to the future balance of the total knee. A more technically demanding aspect of these types of repairs is in the setting of tibial avulsion. Repair in the setting of avulsion has been described with suture anchors or screw and spike washer[8,11,12] (Fig. 5A, B). The repair can be challenging due to the positioning of the bone anchor used to attach the MCL or augment to the femur or tibia. This positioning is critical to provide consistent medial tension throughout the arc of motion, and careful attention must be paid to achieve balance through the range motion. Soft tissue bone anchors are also described for use in setting of avulsion of the periosteum when the MCL proper remains intact.[8] A femoral avulsion of the MCL can be reattached with nonabsorbable sutures secured to the medial femoral condyle through transosseous tunnels or secured with a screw and spiked washer (Fig. 6A–C). With repair of the MCL it may be necessary to increase the level of prosthetic varus/valgus constraint.

Fig. 3. End-to-end repair of lacerated medial collateral ligament (MCL).

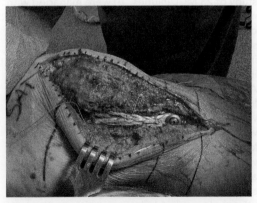

Fig. 4. Repair of the MCL with medial hamstring autograft and semitendinosus allograft. (Photo courtesy of Drs Sam Taylor and Fred Cushner.)

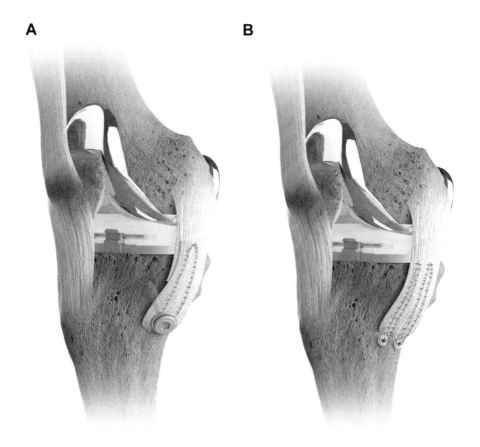

Fig. 5. (*A*) Avulsion of the MCL reattached to tibia with nonabsorbable suture tied over a screw. (*B*) Avulsion of the MCL reattached to tibia with nonabsorbable suture secured to the tibia with suture anchors.

Other authors suggest increasing the constraint level of the implant may be a simpler and more consistent way of managing this issue. Siqueira and colleagues[10] reviewed a series of patients who had intraoperative MCL injury managed with various techniques. In their study of 23 MCL injuries, 10 were managed with no change in implant constraint and had a direct repair, 8 were converted to more constrained implants, 3 received a constrained implant and a repair, and 2 had no change in implant constraint and were left unrepaired. At 5 years postoperatively, these patients had lower overall scores compared to patients with no injury, but between the 4 groups there was no significant difference in outcome or knee function scores. This suggests that repair without constraint and just increasing constraint are both feasible options in this small retrospective study. Caution should be used in situations when considering no repair or increase in constraint. The decision should be based on the level of instability caused by the MCL injury.

Choi and colleagues[11] reviewed patients who had an overrelease of the tibial insertion of the MCL and were repaired with suture anchor. He found no difference in clinical outcomes compared to patients who had no injury in this cohort of patients with posterior stabilized (PS) implants.

Although in many cases simply increasing constraint may be a good option, it is not always a simple conversion. In the setting of a primary CR TKA, conversion to increased constraint is generally more difficult. CR TKA systems have limitations on the ability to convert components to increase varus/valgus constraint. This means that increasing varus/valgus constraint during a CR TKA would require switching components to a PS TKA. Many implant systems use the same tibial component for both systems but do require a change in femoral components. Several major companies have the same internal geometry of the CR and PS femoral component. Since the basic distal femoral bone preparation is the same, conversion to a PS design may be

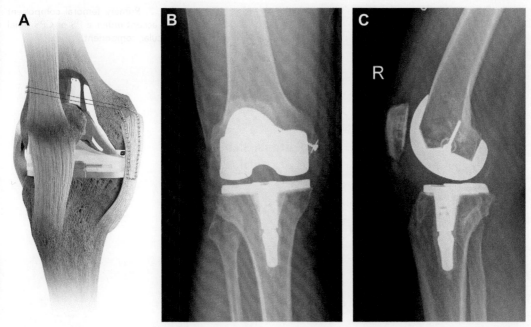

Fig. 6. (A) Avulsion of the MCL reattached to the femur with nonabsorbable suture passed through transosseous tunnels and tied over the lateral femoral cortex. (B, C) AP and lateral radiographs showing avulsion of the MCL reattached to the femur with a screw and spiked washer. The tibial component was a constrained posterior stabilized (CPS) articulation.

as simple as cutting an intercondylar box and inserting the PS tibial articulation.

When the primary implant is a PS TKA construct, several systems allow seamless conversion to a mid-level constraint (MLC) option, without changing implant system at all (Fig. 7). These MLC components allow for increased varus/valgus constraint with primary femoral PS components. These designs have been shown to successfully manage intraoperative instability without affecting clinical outcomes and without increasing any risk of aseptic loosening or causing accelerated wear.[25,26]

The decision to repair, augment, increase constraint, or a combination is multifactorial and depends on the type of implant being used. During CR TKA with a preserved PCL, there is some existing internal medial stability provided by the PCL. In this situation a repair with or without augmentation can provide enough stability to the knee without needing to increase constraint. During a PS TKA with partial MCL injury or overrelease medially, the literature supports increasing constraint to an MLC component. When complete disruption of the MCL occurs MLC implants are not constrained enough to establish stability and in this situation conversion to full varus/valgus constrained knee (CCK) systems is required (Fig. 8). Additionally,

some systems do not have MLC options, which would also require switching to a revision style CCK implant. Hinged knee implants may even be needed in extreme situations with complete loss of medial integrity (Fig. 9). The intricacies of the implant systems and the subtle differences between the components play a major role in successfully managing this predicament. It is critical that surgeons know their primary implant systems' unique features well and have working relationships with their company representatives to assist with options in these situations.

POSTOPERATIVE MANAGEMENT

When more constrained implants are used to manage laxity/injury, there may not be any need to alter postoperative protocols.[4,9] However, in the setting of soft-tissue repair, internal fixation of augmentation, without an increase in constraint, there may be a role for postoperative bracing or immobilization. There are many static and hinged immobilization devices available. The benefits of open style hinged stabilization devices are that the patient may continue with their postoperative rehabilitation and continue to move the knee without restrictions. However, there have been studies, which show that using a hinged

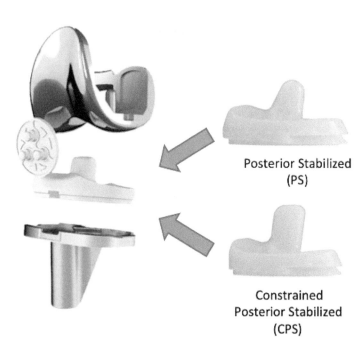

Fig. 7. Primary femoral component can accept either a PS or CPS tibial articular component.

Posterior Stabilized (PS)

Constrained Posterior Stabilized (CPS)

knee brace after TKA with a repaired MCL injury without increasing implant constraint may lead to an increase rate in postoperative stiffness.[14]

There is a wide range of postoperative protocols described in the literature. Lee and Lotke[9] based the postoperative rehabilitation program on the etiology of the injury and how the injury was managed. Patients who were managed with a constrained implant were allowed early motion and immediate full weight bearing without restrictions or brace. Patients who were managed with repair or augmentation of the MCL and had a PS implant were divided into 2 groups: one group was immobilized for 4 weeks prior to initiating their rehabilitation program and the second group had no immobilization and was allowed immediate full weight bearing without restrictions. The authors found, as expected, that all patients had lower overall outcome scores compared to patients without an injury to the MCL, and the patients managed

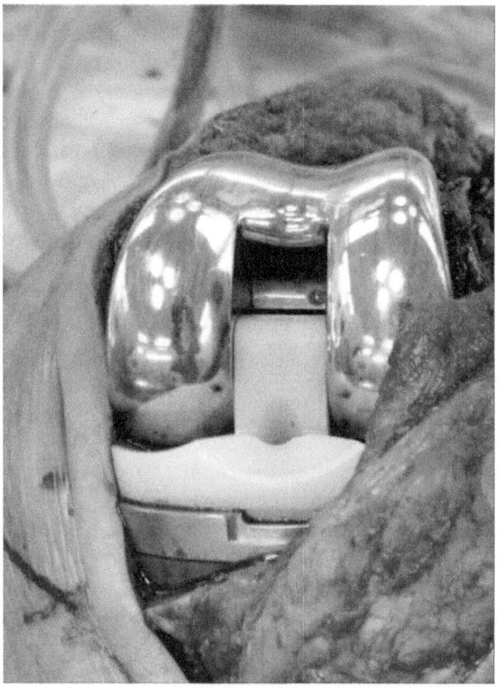

Fig. 8. Constrained condylar knee (CCK) with varus/valgus constraint.

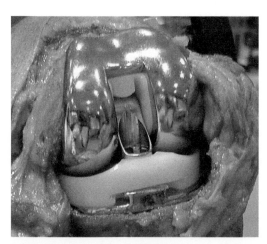

Fig. 9. Rotating hinge knee (RHK).

with a constrained implant had better stability, less revisions for instability, and a better outcome compared to patients managed with MCL repair or augmentation and a less constrained implant.

Leopold and colleagues[8] managed their injuries with direct repair or suture anchor fixation and no change in the type of TKA implanted (12 CR, 4 PS). They braced their patients in a hinged knee brace unlocked for 6 weeks with no reported failures or revisions for instability at 45-month follow-up, with only one case requiring manipulation for stiffness. Shahi and colleagues[12] treated medial instability with synthetic augmented primary repair and maintained a CR TKA using a hinged knee brace for 2 weeks postoperatively. They reported no residual instability in their cohort of 15 patients.

The decision to brace should be made on a case-by-case basis with regard to the type of implant being used, the quality of the repair, and the subjective "feel" of the knee at the end of the surgery. There is a theoretical increased risk of stiffness when postoperative bracing is employed; however, the limited existing literature supports the argument that it may be necessary when preserving CR implants to allow time for the soft tissues to heal. Management of intraoperative medial instability with varus/valgus constraint, with either an MLC for limited instability, CCK for moderate instability, or RHK for severe instability, allows for initiation of postoperative rehabilitation without bracing.

DISCUSSION

The rate of intraoperative medial instability is likely underreported in the literature. Physicians may address these issues intraoperatively and postoperatively without any documentation of iatrogenic injury, by changing their implant choice or using postoperative bracing without any discrete reference as to why those decisions were made. This makes this topic inherently difficult to study and objective data with large cohort numbers difficult to find. The risk factors for medial soft tissue injury are multifactorial and their interplay is complex. Many of the risk factors are potentially avoidable and iatrogenic in nature. A careful examination of the patient preoperatively and reducing any modifiable risk factors may help alleviate the risk. A large factor to this injury, however, is intraoperative and directly related to surgeon experience and skill. Retractor placement and bone resection during TKA has been shown to

have a large learning curve with senior residents graduating from residency in one study still not considered fully proficient in retractor placement during TKA.[27]

Preoperative planning and implant choice can be useful in reducing risk and having alternative options when considering surgery in patients with more severe disease, such as using PS components with options for MLC.

Postoperative Outcomes

Medial instability during TKA can have a profound impact on the outcome when missed or not adequately addressed during primary TKA. Patients with these injuries have worse outcomes compared to matched TKA patients regardless of fixation or treatment technique. Pooled data show significant drops in knee function scores, lower postoperative range of motion, and significantly increased rates of revision and complications.[2] Pooled outcomes presented by Li and colleagues[2] showed more than a 6-fold increased rate of complications and need for revision with complications including instability, aseptic loosening, and infection. These findings reinforce the importance of prevention of MCL injury to reduce the risk of potentially catastrophic complications.

There does not appear to be a consensus in the literature on the best management strategy for intraoperative MCL injury. Regardless of the repair or constraint approach the goal is generally consistent, obtain a TKA, which is balanced medial-lateral and maintains that stability through the arc of motion. Most surgeons appear to lean towards increasing the level of constraint as the most consistent solution with or without repair as the solution to this problem.[9,10,28]

SUMMARY

Maintaining medial stability is critical to a successful TKA regardless of the implant type or system used. Careful attention to the medial soft tissue envelope during TKA will help prevent unnecessary injury and improve patient outcomes from the procedure. An in-depth knowledge of knee anatomy and the use of well-placed retractors will help reduce the risk of injuring the medial side of the knee during TKA. When soft tissue injury does occur, a full evaluation of the injury and treatment with the goal of maintaining stability through the full arch of motion can help prevent poor patient outcomes.

CLINICS CARE POINTS

- Carefully assess the preoperative soft tissue balance before TKA.
- Approach the knee in such a way as to limit unintended overrelease of the medial soft tissues of the knee.
- Take care to place retractors during TKA to protect structures from injury during surgery.
- Assess the integrity of the medial knee soft tissues consistently throughout surgery to allow timely identification of any potential injury.
- Address the injury with either repair, augmentation, or alteration in component constraint, or a combination of these options.
- Assess the integrity and balance of the repair/ alteration prior to completion of the TKA.
- Decide on the necessity of changing postoperative protocols and immobilize or protect with bracing when necessary.
- Management of intraoperative medial instability with varus/valgus constrained implants may be necessary.

DISCLOSURE

The authors have nothing to disclose related to the content of this article.

REFERENCES

1. Sloan M, Premkumar A, Sheth NP. Projected volume of primary total joint arthroplasty in the U.S., 2014 to 2030. J Bone Joint Surg Am 2018;100(17):1455–60.
2. Li J, Yan Z, Lv Y, et al. Impact of intraoperative medial collateral ligament injury on outcomes after total knee arthroplasty: a meta-analysis and systematic review. J Orthop Surg Res 2021;16:686.
3. Whiteside LA. Correction of ligament and bone defects in total arthroplasty of the severely valgus knee. Clin Orthop Relat Res 1993;288:234–45.
4. Koo MH, Choi CH. Conservative treatment for the intraoperative detachment of medial collateral ligament from the tibial attachment site during primary total knee arthroplasty. J Arthroplasty 2009;24(8): 1249–53.
5. Cheung A, Yan CH, Chan PK, et al. The medial collateral ligament in primary total knee arthroplasty: anatomy, biomechanics, and injury. J Am Acad Orthop Surg 2020;28(12):e510–6.
6. Ha CW, Park YB, Lee CH, et al. Selective medial release technique using the pie-crusting method for medial tightness during primary total knee arthroplasty. J Arthroplasty 2016;31(5):1005–10.
7. Dimitris K, Taylor BC, Steensen RN. Excursion of oscillating saw blades in total knee arthroplasty. J Arthroplasty 2010;25(1):158–60.
8. Leopold SS, McStay C, Klafeta K, et al. Primary repair of intraoperative disruption of the medial collateral ligament during total knee arthroplasty. J Bone Jt Surg Am 2001;83(1):86–91.
9. Lee GC, Lotke PA. Management of intraoperative medial collateral ligament injury during TKA. Clin Orthop Relat Res 2011;469(1):64–8.
10. Siqueira MB, Haller K, Mulder A, et al. Outcomes of medial collateral ligament injuries during total knee arthroplasty. J Knee Surg 2016;29(1):68–73.
11. Choi YJ, Lee KW, Seo DK, et al. Conservative management after intraoperative over-release of the medial collateral ligament from its tibial insertion site in patients undergoing total knee arthroplasty. J Knee Surg 2018;31(8):786–91.
12. Shahi A, Tan TL, Tarabichi S, et al. Primary repair of iatrogenic medial collateral ligament injury during TKA: a modified technique. J Arthroplasty 2015; 30(5):854–7.
13. Jung KA, Lee SC, Hwang SH, et al. Quadriceps tendon free graft augmentation for a midsubstance tear of the medial collateral ligament during total knee arthroplasty. Knee 2009;16(6):479–83.
14. Bohl DD, Wetters NG, Del Gaizo DJ, et al. Repair of intraoperative injury to the medial collateral ligament during primary total knee arthroplasty. J Bone Jt Surg Am 2016;98(1):35–9.
15. Canale S.T., Azar F.M., Beaty J.H., et al., Campbell's operative orthopaedics, vol. 3, 13th edition, 2017, Elsevier, Inc.; Philadelphia, 2122–2182, Knee Injuries.
16. LaPrade RF, Engebretsen AH, Ly TV, et al. The anatomy of the medial part of the knee. J Bone Joint Surg 2007;89(9):2000–10.
17. Brantigan OC, Voshell AF. The tibial collateral ligament: its function, its bursae, and its relation to the medial meniscus. J Bone Joint Surg Am 1943;25:121–31.
18. Healy WL, Iorio R, Lemos DW. Medial reconstruction during total knee arthroplasty for severe valgus deformity. Clin Orthop Relat Res 1998; 356:161–9.
19. Winiarsky R, Barth P, Lotke P. Total knee arthroplasty in morbidly obese patients. J Bone Joint Surg Am 1998;80(12):1770–4.
20. Rajkumar N, Soundarrajan D, Dhanasekararaja P, et al. Influence of intraoperative medial collateral ligament bony avulsion injury on the outcome of primary total knee arthroplasty. J Arthroplasty 2021;36(4):1284–94.
21. Scuderi GR, Tenholder M, Capeci C. Surgical approaches in mini-incision total knee arthroplasty. Clin Orthop Relat Res 2004;428:61–7.

22. Shah N, Nilesh G, Patel N. Mini-subvastus approach for total knee arthroplasty in obese patients. Indian J Orthop 2010;44(3):292–9.

23. Hampp EL, Sodhi N, Scholl L, et al. Less iatrogenic soft-tissue damage utilizing robotic-assisted total knee arthroplasty when compared with a manual approach: a blinded assessment. Bone Joint Res 2019;8(10):495–501.

24. Kitamura N, Ogawa M, Kondo E, et al. A novel medial collateral ligament reconstruction procedure using semitendinosus tendon autograft in patients with multiligamentous knee injuries: clinical outcomes. Am J Sports Med 2013;41(6): 1274–81.

25. Crawford DA, Law JI, Lombardi AV Jr, et al. Midlevel constraint without stem extensions in primary total knee arthroplasty provides stability without compromising fixation. J Arthroplasty 2018;33(9): 2800–3.

26. Yohe N, Vanderbrook DJ, Sherman AE, et al. Stability with a Constrained Posterior Stabilized Primary Total Knee Arthroplasty Does Not Compromise Durability. J Knee Surg 2023;36(8): 801–5.

27. Harper KD, Brown LD, Lambert BS, et al. Technical obstacles in total knee arthroplasty learning: a steps breakdown evaluation. JAAOS: Global Research and Reviews 2019;3(6). e19.00062.

28. Dragosloveanu S, Cristea S, Stoica C, et al. Outcome of iatrogenic collateral ligaments injuries during total knee arthroplasty. Eur J Orthop Surg Traumatol 2014;24:1499–503.

Trauma

Intraoperative Imaging Challenges During Pelvic Ring Disruptions and Acetabular Fracture Surgery

Ian G. Hasegawa, MD[a], Joshua L. Gary, MD[a,*]

KEYWORDS

- Radiograph • Computer tomography • Fluoroscopic imaging • Pelvic ring • Acetabulum

---

KEY POINTS

- Early identification of patient obesity, excessive bowel gas, abdominal/pelvic packing, and contrast dye on preoperative plain radiographs can mitigate imaging challenges that may develop during surgery.
- Preoperative computer tomography studies, including three-dimensional reformatted sequences, can be used to anticipate intraoperative image angles, identify sacral dysmorphism, and define fracture planes and displacements in a similar manner as will be observed during surgery.
- Operating room setup, fluoroscopic equipment, and consistent use of instructional terminology help facilitate effective and efficient fluoroscopy workflow.

INTRODUCTION

Intraoperative imaging, most commonly via fluoroscopy, plays an important role in the successful surgical management of pelvic ring disruptions and acetabular fractures. It is the primary method in which clamp placement, reduction accuracy, and implant positioning are assessed. Intraoperative fluoroscopy is also routinely used to evaluate occult pelvic ring instability.[1] Technological advancements in intraoperative fluoroscopy have expanded the indications for percutaneous fixation of the pelvic ring and acetabulum. Some injuries that were previously treated with open approaches can now be reduced and stabilized using minimal incisions. The benefits of percutaneous fixation are multifactorial, including decreased blood loss, surgical time, wound complications, hospital stay, heterotopic ossification formation, and nonunion.[2]

However, obtaining clear and reliable intraoperative fluoroscopic images can be technically challenging. A complete understanding of the osteology and radiographic anatomy of the pelvic ring and acetabulum, including normal variations in sacral morphology, is mandatory. A single-view image is insufficient to accurately and reliably define reduction quality, osseous fixation pathways, and implant positioning. Instead, multiple images obtained in multiple planes are needed. Image angles must also be precise and reproducible; otherwise, misinterpretation can ensue. Fluoroscopic image quality can be compromised by patient positioning, body habitus, bowel gas, contrast dye, and equipment limitations. Fracture malreduction, errant implant placement, and neurovascular injury have all been attributed to inadequate intraoperative fluoroscopic imaging.[3–5]

The purpose of this article is to review common intraoperative imaging challenges during pelvic ring and acetabular fracture fixation surgery. Additionally, practical tips and evidence-

---

[a] Keck School of Medicine of USC, 1520 San Pablo Street. HC2 – Suite 2000, Los Angeles, CA 90033, USA
* Corresponding author. Department of Orthopaedic Surgery, Keck School of Medicine of USC, 1520 San Pablo Street, Suite 2000, Los Angeles, CA 90033.
E-mail address: Joshua.Gary@med.usc.edu

Orthop Clin N Am 55 (2024) 73–87
https://doi.org/10.1016/j.ocl.2023.07.004
0030-5898/24/© 2023 Elsevier Inc. All rights reserved.

based intraoperative imaging strategies will be discussed.

PREOPERATIVE PLANNING

A thoughtful preoperative plan is the first step toward achieving effective and efficient intraoperative fluoroscopy and may mitigate some of the frequently encountered challenges with imaging quality. The preoperative plan should include a careful evaluation of plain radiographs and computer tomography (CT) scans, including three-dimensional (3D) reconstruction images, to identify barriers to quality fluoroscopic imaging, measure anticipated image angles, and gain a better understanding of the patient-specific osteology, fracture planes, and displacements.

Pelvic ring disruptions and acetabular fractures frequently occur in polytraumatized patients. Although necessary, many of the nonorthopedic procedures and treatments that are performed acutely can compromise intraoperative fluoroscopic image quality. Excessive bowel gas accumulation, contrast dye, abdominal or pelvic packing, and wound vacuums are easily identified on preoperative plain radiographs (Fig. 1). A foley catheter is recommended for every pelvic and acetabular case and is also helpful for decompressing bladder contrast. Oral contrast agents should be avoided before surgery since bowel contrast is much more difficult to remedy. Abdominal or pelvic packing and wound vacuums, under most circumstances, can be removed before fracture fixation but should be coordinated with the general surgery team. Excessive bowel gas accumulation, in some cases, can make it impossible to reliably delineate the sacral foramina on intraoperative fluoroscopy. Nitrous oxide anesthesia has been associated with bowel gas accumulation and therefore should be avoided.[6] To improve image quality in the setting of excessive bowel gas shadows, Patel and colleagues suggests combining fluoroscopy beam collimation to improve image contrast with abdominal massage to manually displace gas shadows away from sacral neuroforamina.[7]

Obesity and morbid obesity pose significant challenges to obtaining high-quality intraoperative images during the surgical fixation of pelvic ring disruptions and acetabular fractures. The dense fat envelope attenuates fluoroscopic beam penetration and increases photon scatter resulting in low contrast, less-defined images (see Fig. 1).[8] Inlet and outlet tilt angles are physically restricted by the patient's abdominal and thigh girth. Often a view of the entire pelvic

ring is not attainable in a single image because the image intensifier cannot be lowered sufficiently. Miller and colleagues found a high correlation between preoperative lateral scout CT and intraoperative fluoroscopic images in morbidly obese patients.[9] Specifically, when the lateral sacrum is not visualized on a preoperative scout CT, a reliable true lateral view of the sacrum cannot be obtained on intraoperative fluoroscopy. From a practical standpoint, mobilization of the abdominal pannus away from the image field with foam or silk tape before sterile prep and draping may be helpful. Additionally, increasing the peak kilovoltage and using bucky grids can improve beam penetration and reduce image scatter, respectively.[8] These methods, however, will also increase radiation exposure to both patient and surgeon.[10] Beam collimation or coning is a useful technique for reducing the radiation dose while simultaneously increasing image contrast.

Biplanar and triplanar intraoperative fluoroscopy is needed to achieve reductions and place implants safely through the bony corridors of the pelvic ring and acetabulum. The various images include the anterior posterior (AP) pelvis, inlet, outlet, lateral sacral, obturator oblique (OO), iliac oblique (IO), and combined obturator oblique outlet (COOO) and combined obturator oblique inlet (COOI) views (Table 1). The technical aspects for achieving these views and interpreting their findings have been well described.[11]

Various studies demonstrate the benefits of preoperative two-dimensional (2D) CT scans for anticipating intraoperative fluoroscopic view angles. Traditionally, inlet and outlet images are obtained by tilting the fluoroscopy beam 45° in the cranial and caudal direction, respectively. Multiple studies have since demonstrated that inlet and outlet angles are not orthogonal.[12–14] Eastman and Rout describe using a line drawn parallel to the anterior cortex of the S1 body and a line overlying the pubic symphysis to the center of the S2 body on a midsagittal CT reconstruction view for determining ideal inlet and outlet views, respectively (Fig. 2).[14] In their series, the average ideal inlet angle was 25° and the ideal outlet angle was 42°. This differed from the measured intraoperative fluoroscopic inlet and outlet angles by 4.4° and 0.45°, respectively. The authors thus concluded that intraoperative fluoroscopic inlet and outlet angles could be anticipated within 5° of preoperative CT measurements. Importantly, Ricci and colleagues demonstrated that ideal inlet and outlet angles can differ considerably between S1 and S2 bodies.[12] Therefore, a single tilt angle may

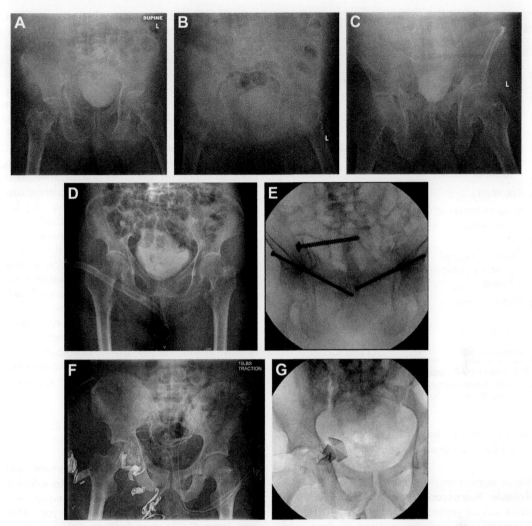

Fig. 1. Examples of barriers to optimal intraoperative imaging seen on preoperative plain radiographs. A 63-year-old man with a right anterior column posterior hemitransverse acetabular fracture (A–C). Preoperative AP, inlet and outlet radiographs with poor image quality due to patient's obesity, bladder contrast, and poor bone quality. A 92-year-old female with an unstable lateral compression type 1 pelvic ring injury (D, E). Preoperative AP radiograph with poor image quality due to excessive bowel gasses and bladder contrast (D) and intraoperative fluoroscopic outlet image of the same patient demonstrating difficult visualization of the S1 neuroforamen (E). A 48-year-old man with a lateral compression type 3 pelvic ring injury. Preoperative AP pelvis radiograph demonstrating abdominal and pelvic packing near the right pubic root (F). Intraoperative fluoroscopic AP pelvis image demonstrating incomplete visualization of the right pubic root and acetabulum (G).

not be reliable for placing iliosacral screws at multiple upper sacral levels (Fig. 3). Axial CT images are also useful for planning ideal oblique image angles (see Fig. 2).

The normal sagittal alignment of the sacrum can vary widely between patients and because of traumatic injury, such as with spinopelvic dissociation (Fig. 4).[15,16] This can be easily observed on preoperative sagittal CT imaging. Because of this, the angles needed to obtain reliable inlet and outlet views intraoperatively will also vary widely. Ricci and colleagues describe

the ideal outlet view as perpendicular to the upper sacral segment body.[12] This makes achieving reliable outlet views difficult in the setting of increased upper sacral flexion, as commonly seen in a spinopelvic dissociation. The vertical orientation of a flexed sacrum when supine requires a high outlet tilt angle to achieve a reliable image. In some instances, this can exceed the C-arm clearance as the patient's body or undersurface of the table interferes with higher tilt angles. We have found that positioning a sacral bump more distally under the patient to extend

Table 1
Injury location/fixation pathway and fluoroscopy view

Injury location/ Fixation Pathway	Fluoroscopy View
Pubic symphysis	Inlet and outlet
Supra-acetabular, LC2	COO, IO, COI, and lateral sacral
Gluteal pillar, iliac crest external fixation	IO and OO
Iliac crest	IO, OO, COOI
Iliosacral/transiliac transsacral	Inlet, hyperinlet, outlet, COOI, and lateral sacral
Anterior column/ superior pubic ramus	COO and inlet
Posterior column	AP, IO, and lateral sacral
Anterior wall	OO and IO
Posterior wall	OO and IO

Abbreviations: AP, anterior posterior pelvis; COO, combined obturator oblique; COOI, combined obturator oblique inlet; IO, iliac oblique; OO, obturator oblique.

the sacrum can help decrease the necessary outlet tilt to an unobstructed range.

Three-dimensional Reconstructions

Reliable fluoroscopic imaging of dysmorphic sacra can be particularly challenging to obtain. Pekmezci and colleagues used surface and volume-rendered 3D CT images to recreate the "perfect" inlet and outlet view in dysmorphic and nondysmorphic sacra.[17] Each 3D image of the pelvis was rotated around a vertical axis in 1° increments until an ideal inlet and outlet image was obtained. The ideal inlet view was defined when the sacral promontory overlapped the anterior cortex of S1, and the ideal outlet view was defined when the pubic symphysis was superimposed over the S2 body (Fig. 5). In dysmorphic sacra, the ideal inlet view was achieved with 25° of caudal tilt, and the ideal outlet view was achieved with 43° of cranial tilt. The authors also found good correlation between surface-rendered and volume-rendered CT images. Inlet angles between dysmorphic and nondysmorphic sacra were similar, whereas dysmorphic sacral required on average an additional 5° of cranial tilt. Conflitti and colleagues correlated the findings of preoperative 3D surface-rendered and volume-rendered CT

images with intraoperative fluoroscopy when placing S2 transsacral screws in dysmorphic sacra.[18] In this study, the authors demonstrated that 3D CT reconstruction images highlight the anterior cortical indentations of the upper sacral segment alar zones on an inlet view, and the steep medial to lateral alar slopes on an outlet view. Twenty of 24 patients demonstrated complete intraosseous screw placement, whereas 4 of 24 patients had juxtaforaminal screws.

Three-dimensional CT reconstruction also plays an important role in the preoperative planning of acetabular fractures. Fracture planes, displacements, and spatial orientations can be studied on perfect AP, judet, inlet, outlet, and lateral sacral views. Additionally, femoral head subtraction allows for the direct visualization of articular fracture lines. This information is vital for planning reduction maneuvers, fixation constructs, and implant placement because it will be seen on intraoperative fluoroscopic images. Scott and colleagues reviewed the preoperative plain radiographs, 2D CT scans, and 3D CT reconstruction images of 40 acetabular fractures.[19] Review of the 3D surface-rendered images resulted in a change in surgical approach and treatment in 30% of cases.

EQUIPMENT, SETUP, AND COMMUNICATION

Having the right fluoroscopy equipment and operating room (OR) setup is key to efficient fluoroscopy workflow. The basic equipment needed includes a radiolucent flat top table and large C-arm that facilitates unobstructed clearance of the OR table, table attachments, patient, and surgical instruments. The OR should be large enough to allow easy side-to-side transitions between the C-arm machine and sterile back table when bilateral fixation is needed. A 12″ image intensifier (or larger) is ideal so that a view of the entire pelvic ring can be obtained in a single image. This will be helpful for judging symmetry and trajectories, such as during transsacral-transiliac screw placement. Flat panel image intensifiers, compared with circular, are associated with less image distortion secondary to parallax but are not mandatory.[20] In general, targeting the focal point of the image centrally in the image field minimizes the effective parallax.[21] Most modern C-arms have a roll over the top range from 25° to 55°. A higher roll over the top range provides greater versatility for obtaining oblique images. The basic fluoroscopy setup consists of the C-arm stationed opposite from the surgeon with the

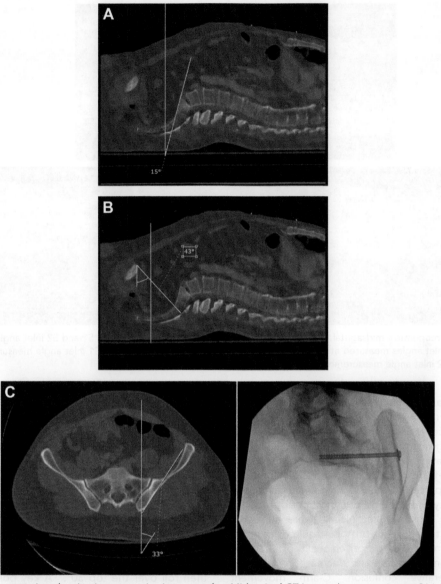

Fig. 2. Preoperative planning intraoperative image angles. Midsagittal CT image demonstrating an S1 inlet angle measurement of 15° (A). Midsagittal CT image demonstrating an outlet angle measurement of 43° (B). Axial CT image at S1 demonstrating an obturator rollover angle measurement of 33° (C) and the corresponding COOI intra-operative fluoroscopic image. COOI, combined obturator oblique inlet.

base oriented perpendicular to the patient. When imaging, the C-arm should be positioned centrally over the pelvis or hip in such a way that biplanar imaging can be repeated with min-imal translation of the C-arm base. Tilt angles and base positions should be marked for more efficient transition in and out with the C-arm. Cords and lines should be secured outside of the image field and not impede movements of the C-arm base or gantry. Similarly, the surgeon should have an easy unobstructed view of the fluoroscopy monitor. Typically, the monitor is

stationed at the foot of the bed. Patient posi-tioning devices and table attachments can also compromise fluoroscopic image quality. This in-cludes sacral bumps, chest rolls, traction attach-ments, and arm board holders among others (Fig. 6). We have found using folded blankets as sacral bumps and rolled blankets for chest rolls to be less radiopaque compared with sheets and gel pads. All unnecessary table at-tachments should be removed.

The benefits of establishing clear and consistent communication between surgeon and radiology

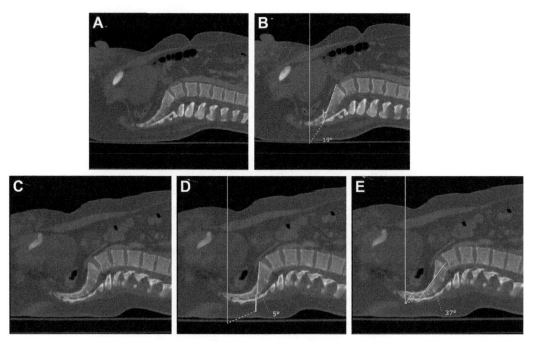

Fig. 3. Preoperative midsagittal CT S1 and S2 inlet angle measurements. Colinear S1 and S2 inlet angles (A). S1 and S2 inlet angles measured at 19° (B). Noncolinear S1 and S2 inlet angles (C). S1 inlet angle measurement of 5° (D). S2 inlet angle measurement of 37° (E).

technician have been well documented. The use of common fluoroscopic language has been shown to reduce fluoroscopy time as well as the number of images taken.[22–24] Burke and colleagues investigated the effects of a standardized intraoperative fluoroscopy language education protocol on the perceived quality of communication and efficiency in the OR.[24] Forty orthopedic surgeons and 41 radiology technicians were surveyed. Overall, the education protocol resulted in a significant increase in the perceived quality of intraoperative communication and decrease in perceived intraoperative confusion, C-arm movement corrections, and need for repeat fluoroscopic

images. Mean fluoroscopy time also significantly decreased after the education protocol (90 + 106 seconds vs 52.7 + 39.2 seconds, $P < .004$).

Instructions should be communicated to the radiology technician in a systematic fashion beginning with the specific C-arm movement, followed by the direction, and quantification of the desired movement (Table 2). When a combination of movements is needed, distinct instructions should be given for each movement. For example, "Tilt toward the head 25°, then roll over the top 30°." A key point when transitioning between views, consideration

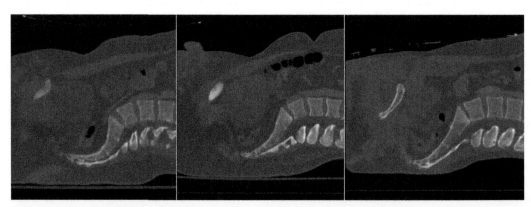

Fig. 4. Variations in sagittal sacral alignment.

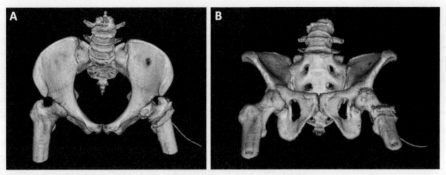

Fig. 5. Ideal inlet (A) and outlet (B) 3D surface-rendered image views.

should be given to the movement sequence that allows the C-arm to move/rotate around the surgeon and surgical instruments, rather than the surgeon around the C-arm. This allows the surgeon to maintain important reductions, start points, and trajectories throughout the image sequence.

POSTERIOR PELVIC RING

As previously discussed, the preoperative planning is critical to success with posterior fixation in the pelvic ring. One thing the surgeon must remember is that manipulative reduction maneuvers, closed or open, may change the osseous

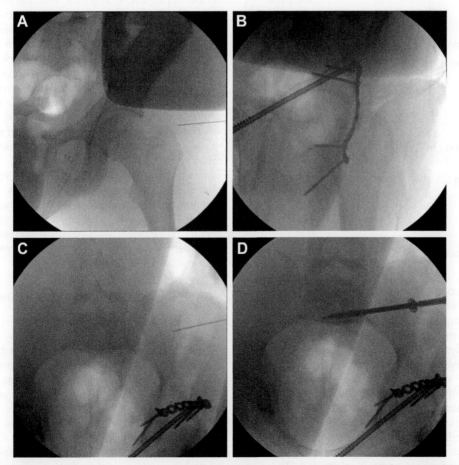

Fig. 6. 17 year-old male patient with a combined left transverse posterior wall acetabular fracture and ipsilateral incomplete sacroiliac joint injury placed in the prone position. Gel pad chest rolls creating radiopaque shadows over the supra-acetabular (A, B) and sacral alar (C, D) regions.

Table 2
C-arm movements, terminology, and direction

C-arm Movement	Terminology	Direction
Arm driven		
Raise and lower	Raise Lower	Up Down
In and out	Push in Pull out	Toward "me" Toward "you"
Cant	Tilt	Toward the head (ie, Inlet) Toward the feet (ie, Outlet)
Axial rotation	Roll Orbit "C"	Over (the top) Under
Wag	Wig wag	Toward the head (ie, Proximal) Toward the feet (ie, Distal)
Base driven		
Slide	Slide	Toward the head (ie, Proximal) Toward the feet (ie, Distal)
In and out	Push in Pull out	Toward "me" Toward "you"
Wag	Wig wag	Toward the head (ie, Proximal) Toward the feet (ie, Distal)

fixation pathways visualized on preoperative imaging and anticipated angles required for visualization.

For the upper sacral segment, identifying sacral dysmorphism is critical to safely place implants without causing damage to the L4, L5, and S1 nerve roots. Preoperative 3D surface-rendered reconstruction views allow the surgeon to visualize the "indentation" in the upper sacral segment that is visualized on an inlet image (Fig. 7). By ensuring all instrumentation remains posterior to indentation, risk of damage to the L4 and L5 nerve roots is minimized. The first implant in an iliosacral vector should be placed in a low and anterior position in the upper sacral

segment as positions too cranial on an outlet image risk damage to L4 and L5 nerve roots unless the implant is cranial and posterior. When a cranial and posterior implant is chosen, frequent with multiple screws in the upper sacral segment, it is important to establish the posterior limits of the sacral osseous fixation pathway. Although the traditional inlet view establishes the anterior cortical limit of the sacrum, it does not provide a reliable view of the posterior cortical limit. The "hyperinlet" images, as described by Gosselin and colleagues, add additional inlet tilt to a traditional inlet view in order to delineate the anterior border of the sacral canal.[25] This can be measured preoperatively on a midsagittal CT scan by defining the angle formed by a vertical line and one that parallels the posterior aspect of S1 (Fig. 8). In their case series, the additional inlet tilt required to achieve a hyperinlet view averaged 17°.

For patients without sacral dysmorphism, transsacral-transiliaic (TSTI) vectors can be used in the upper sacral segment and the anterior cortical limits of the upper and second sacral segments are usually collinear. The "hyperinlet" image is useful when 2 screws are placed in a TSTI pathway, with one screw low and anterior and the second screw cranial and posterior (Fig. 9). Fixation in the second sacral segment may be safely placed just posterior to the anterior cortex of the sacrum on an inlet radiograph and at the junction of a line dividing the middle and caudal thirds of the space between the S1 and S2 foramina on the outlet image (see Fig. 8).

In a patient with sacral dysmorphism, implant placement should be done in the upper sacral segment before the second sacral segment because an implant in proper position in the second sacral segment will prevent visualization of the indentation in the upper sacral segment on inlet imaging (see Fig. 8).

ANTERIOR COLUMN/SUPERIOR PUBIC RAMUS

Percutaneous anterior column/superior pubic ramus intramedullary fixation remains a technically challenging skill for many surgeons. The combination of fluoroscopic views that most accurately and reliably demonstrate the cortical limits of the anterior column/superior pubic ramus osseous fixation pathway has been debated. Traditionally, pelvic inlet and COOO views have been used to assess the anterior-posterior and cranial-caudal cortical limits, respectively.[11] More recently, additional views have been recommended.[26–28] Cunningham

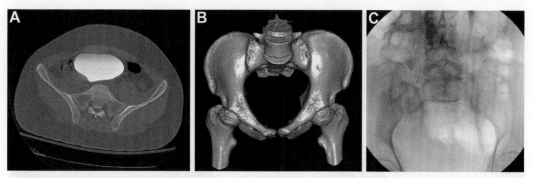

Fig. 7. Axial and inlet views of a dysmorphic sacrum. Axial CT image at S1 (*A*), 3D surface-rendered CT inlet image (*B*) and intraoperative fluoroscopic inlet image (*C*). Note the easy visualization of the sacral alar indentations on the 3D surface-rendered CT image.

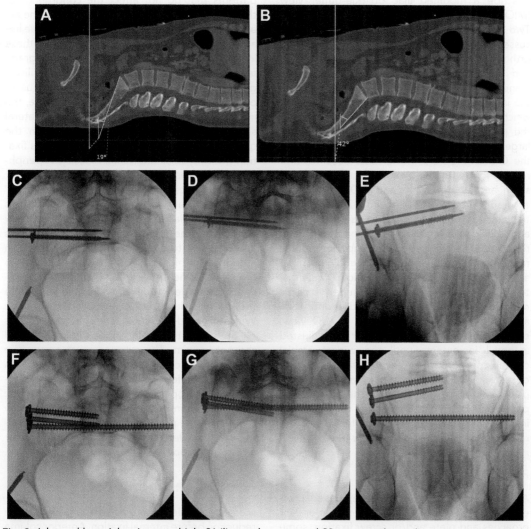

Fig. 8. Inlet and hyperinlet views, multiple S1 iliosacral screws, and S2 transsacral transiliac screw. A 46-year-old man with a lateral compression type 3 pelvic ring injury. Preoperative midsagittal CT inlet angle measurement of 19° (*A*) and hyperinlet angle measurement of 42° (*B*). Intraoperative fluoroscopic inlet (*C, F*) and hyperinlet (*D, G*) images. Caudal anterior and cranial posterior S1 iliosacral screw positioning (*C–H*). Well-positioned S2 transsacral transiliac screw placed after S1 iliosacral screws.

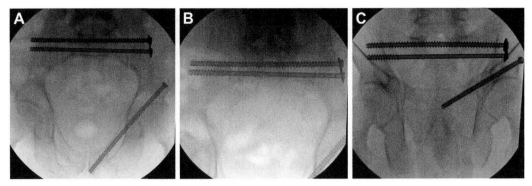

Fig. 9. Two transsacral transiliac screw in S1 with a low and anterior and cranial and posterior screw in the corridor. (*A*) Inlet (*B*) Hyperinlet (*C*) Outlet views after screw placement.

describe a modified iliac oblique-outlet view (MIOO) as an alternative to the pelvic inlet.[26] Two distinct advantages of the MIOO were discussed. First, the MIOO and COOO views are orthogonal. This facilitates C-arm, start point and trajectory adjustments to occur in one plane. Second, the MIOO is easily obtained in the lateral position, unlike the pelvic inlet view, which is often obstructed by arm boards and the patient's body, particularly if they are of large habits. Guimaraes and colleagues found the OO and COOO views most accurate and reliable for determining extra-articular screw position, and the pelvic inlet and MIOO views most accurate and reliable for intraosseous positioning.[29] It is our practice to use pelvic inlet and COOO views when placing antegrade or retrograde anterior column/superior pubic ramus screws. Similar to Bishop and Routt, we aim to achieve an inlet beam angle tangential to the posterior cortex of the superior pubic ramus, such that the superior and inferior rami are not superimposed.[11] On the COOO view, outlet tilt and obturator roll over are adjusted in small increments until the widest cranial caudal corridor at the acetabular isthmus is observed. Ideal positioning of intramedullary implants should be tangential to the apex of the posterior border of the superior ramus on the inlet view and above the acetabulum and obturator foramen on the COOO view (**Fig. 10**).

POSTERIOR COLUMN

Although many posterior column injuries are preferentially stabilized with open posterior approaches and plate and/or screw fixation, some fracture patterns may be amenable to percutaneous or columnar fixation of the posterior column. These often include minimally displaced fracture or more caudal transverse fracture patterns that do not affect the congruency of the cranial femoral head and the dome of the acetabulum. The AP (or outlet) and iliac oblique images are used for the placement of these implants, which can be placed in an antegrade fashion (through the lateral window of the ilioinguinal approach) or in a retrograde fashion using percutaneous techniques. On the AP image, the implant should be just lateral to the quadrilateral surface. Screws directed peripheral from the quadrilateral surface often exit the osseous fixation pathway near the ischial recess just peripheral to the lesser sciatic notch. An obturator outlet image can be used in addition to the AP (or outlet) view to visualize an extraosseous implant. The iliac oblique view ensures the screw is anterior to the greater and lesser sciatic notches and posterior to the joint. Implants placed in an antegrade fashion usually terminate just distal to the ischial spine because the rib cage often prevents the surgeon from directing the implant to the most caudal aspect of the ischial tuberosity. With retrograde placement, the implant begins on the ischial tuberosity and is directed toward the pelvic brim. The surgeon must ensure the screw is not too long into the iliacus fossa. A lateral sacral view can aid the surgeon in determining the proper ending point of a retrograde posterior column screw. The iliac cortical density represents the pelvic brim and provides the surgeon an excellent marker of a safe endpoint for a retrograde posterior column screw (**Fig. 11**).

ACETABULAR FRACTURES

Most acetabular fractures will undergo open reduction before internal fixation. Anterior column screws are commonly placed using fluoroscopic guidance for fractures in transverse-family when a Kocher-Langenbeck approach is chosen. Fluoroscopic imaging should be used to confirm that all

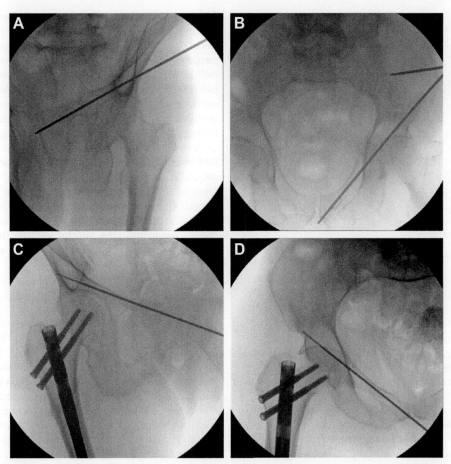

Fig. 10. Well-positioned antegrade guidewire placement on COOO and inlet views (A, B). Well-positioned retrograde drill bit placement on COOO and inlet views (C, D). COOO, combined obturator oblique outlet.

implants are extra-articular during the surgery because only one image demonstrating a screw is extra-articular is needed to confirm the absence of intra-articular implants. Several studies have investigated the optimal view for determining extra-articular screw placement. Norris and colleagues demonstrated that any one view of the acetabulum demonstrating separation between screw and articular surface is sufficient to confirm extra-articular positioning.[30] In their study, a true lateral view of the pelvis was found to be most accurate for determining extra-articular position of posteriorly based screws. Axial or "on end" fluoroscopic views have been shown to be equivalent to postoperative CT for detecting intra-articular screw positioning in patients operated on in the lateral position.[31,32] This view typically requires iliac oblique rotation and varying degrees of inlet or outlet tilt until an on end view of the screw head is achieved.[32] For acetabular fracture surgery done prone, Tosoundidis and colleagues demonstrated the effectiveness of a combined inlet obturator oblique view for extra-articular placement of

posterior wall lag screws.[33] Regardless of patient position, Wu and colleagues demonstrated that peripheral-based posterior wall plate screws along the lateral brim are at the highest risk for intra-articular penetration.[34] Therefore, because the screw entry point along the posterior wall shifts from medial to peripheral, greater screw angulation is needed to avoid penetrating the joint.

INTRAOPERATIVE COMPUTER TOMOGRAPHY

There are times during pelvic ring and acetabular fracture surgery when intraoperative fluoroscopy, despite all attempts, is insufficient to accurately and reliably confirm reduction quality and implant position. Additionally, in certain patients, there is little correlation between preoperative and intraoperative image findings. For example, circumferential compression devices placed before preoperative CT imaging have the potential to mask or accentuate pelvic ring injury severity.[35] Additionally, preoperative CT

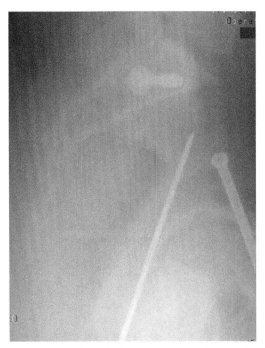

Fig. 11. Lateral sacral view of a retrograde posterior column screw with the screw tip positioned caudal to the pelvic brim.

imaging of fracture dislocations are sometimes performed in an unreduced state without repeat imaging obtained after closed reduction attempts and before surgery. In these situations, surgeons are required to make important intraoperative decisions based on suboptimal information. This can place patients at risk for inadequate reductions, misplaced implants, and revision surgeries.[36]

Multiple studies investigating the utility of advanced intraoperative imaging during pelvic ring and acetabular fracture surgery have been undertaken. Acetabular fracture fixation and iliosacral screw placement under CT image guidance has been associated with improved quality of reduction and screw positioning.[37–39] In contrast, other authors have found no differences regarding screw positioning when comparing computer-navigated and conventional fluoroscopic guided iliosacral screw placement.[40] Although the results of this study may have been influenced by surgeon experience.

Intraoperative multidimensional fluoroscopy (IMF) using the Ziehm Vision RFD 3D (Ziehm Nuremburg, Germany) has become popularized during the recent years. Shaw and colleagues reported on 52 cases of unstable posterior pelvic ring disruptions.[41] Guide pin insertion for percutaneous iliosacral or transiliac transsacral screw fixation was performed under traditional fluoroscopy. IMF was then obtained after screw fixation. No screws were found to be intraforaminal on IMF or postoperative CT. Forty-two percent of patients received more than one IMF spin, 5 patients received IMF before guide pin placement to assess the available bony corridor after a reduction maneuver, 3 patients underwent IMF after guide pin insertion but before definitive screw fixation, and 2 patients underwent screw revision after reviewing the IMF findings. Routt and colleagues reported on several cases where IMF was helpful for identifying retained intra-articular loose bodies, malreduced dome comminution, and misdirected screws.[36] Additionally, specific mention was made regarding the usefulness of IMF in morbidly obese patients and combined acetabular pelvic ring injuries.

SUMMARY

Obtaining clear and reliable intraoperative images during pelvic ring and acetabular fracture fixation surgery is challenging due to the complex osteology and injury patterns involved, as well as the unique characteristics of each patient and the technical demands of the procedure. A meticulous and comprehensive preoperative plan can help anticipate and mitigate many of these challenges, thereby preventing them from devloping during the surgery. Preoperative plain radiographs offer valuable insight into potential challenges that can compromise intraoperative image quality, such as body habitus, bowel gases, contrast dye, and abdominal packing. These factors can be identified and addressed before surgery to ensure optimal imaging intraoperatively. Preoperative CT studies provide an opportunity to proactively anticipate image angles and gain a deeper understanding of the osteology and bony displacements because they will be seen intraoperatively. It is essential not to overlook the significance of appropriate fluoroscopy equipment, room setup, and consistent communication between the surgeon and radiology technician. These factors play a crucial role in ensuring the effectiveness of intraoperative imaging and promoting efficient workflow. When achieving high-quality intraoperative imaging is not possible, advanced imaging techniques such as CT and multidimensional fluoroscopy can be highly effective. The information provided by these specialty devices may eliminate uncertainty of safe screw corridors and appropriate reduction while reducing unnecessary secondary surgeries by identifying problems in real time.

CLINICS CARE POINTS

- Suboptimal intraoperative fluoroscopic imaging can lead to fracture malreduction, errant implant placement, and neurovascular injury.[3–5]

- When excessive bowel gas is present, image quality can be improved with abdominal massage to displace bowel gases away from sacral neuroformina and beam collimation to enhance image contrast.[7]

- In morbidly obese patients, a reliable lateral sacral fluoroscopic image is unachievable when the lateral sacrum cannot be visualized on a preoperative lateral scout CT image.[9]

- Inlet and outlet image angles are nonorthogonal and can be anticipated with reasonable accuracy when measured on preoperative midsagittal CT scans.[14]

- Inlet and outlet image angles will vary widely between patients due to the wide range of sagittal sacral tilt present.[15]

- Standardized fluoroscopy language can improve OR communication and fluoroscopy efficiency.[24]

- When multiple or a cranial posterior iliosacral screw is planned, a hyperinlet view is useful for delineating the posterior cortical limit of the upper sacral segments.[25]

- The modified iliac oblique outlet view is an alternative view for determining accurate and safe positioning of anterior column/superior pubic ramus screws.[26]

- Extra-articular screw positioning during acetabular fixation can be confirmed with a single view demonstrating separation between the articular surface and implant.[30]

- IMF is a useful tool for confirming reduction accuracy and safe implant placement when optimal intraoperative imaging is unachievable.[41]

DISCLOSURE

I.G. Hasegawa has nothing to disclose. J.L. Gary has something to disclose. Detailed relevant disclosure information is available at AAOS.org/disclosure.

REFERENCES

1. Sagi HC, Coniglione FM, Stanford JH. Examination under anesthetic for occult pelvic ring instability. J Orthop Trauma 2011;25(9). https://doi.org/10.1097/BOT.0b013e31822b02ae.

2. Giannoudis PV, Tzioupis CC, Pape HC, et al. Percutaneous fixation of the pelvic ring. Journal of Bone and Joint Surgery - Series B 2007;89(2). https://doi.org/10.1302/0301-620X.89B2.18551.

3. Routt MLC. Iliosacral screw fixation: Early complications of the percutaneous technique. J Orthop Trauma 1997;11(8). https://doi.org/10.1097/00005131-199711000-00007.

4. Banaszek D, Starr AJ, Lefaivre KA. Technical Considerations and Fluoroscopy in Percutaneous Fixation of the Pelvis and Acetabulum. J Am Acad Orthop Surg 2019;27(24). https://doi.org/10.5435/JAAOS-D-18-00102.

5. Hadeed M, Heare A, Parry J, et al. Anatomical Considerations in Percutaneous Fixation of the Pelvis and Acetabulum. J Am Acad Orthop Surg 2021;29(19). https://doi.org/10.5435/jaaos-d-21-00066.

6. Bates P, Gary J, Singh G, et al. Percutaneous treatment of pelvic and acetabular fractures in obese patients. Orthop Clin N Am 2011;42(1). https://doi.org/10.1016/j.ocl.2010.08.004.

7. Patel S, Dhillon M, Vashisht S, et al. Pinhole effect and manual bowel gas displacement: Simple two tricks for better fluoroscopy imaging in iliosacral screw fixation. Journal of Orthopaedic Diseases and Traumatology 2020;3(1). https://doi.org/10.4103/jodp.jodp_3_20.

8. Uppot RN. Impact of Obesity on Radiology. Radiol Clin North Am 2007;45(2). https://doi.org/10.1016/j.rcl.2007.03.001.

9. Miller AN, Krieg JC, Routt ML. Lateral Sacral Imaging in the Morbidly Obese. J Orthop Trauma 2013;27(5). https://doi.org/10.1097/BOT.0b013e31826046b0.

10. Yanch JC, Behrman RH, Hendricks MJ, et al. Increased radiation dose to overweight and obese patients from radiographic examinations. Radiology 2009;252(1). https://doi.org/10.1148/radiol.2521080141.

11. Bishop JA, Routt ML, Chip). Osseous fixation pathways in pelvic and acetabular fracture surgery. J Trauma Acute Care Surg 2012;72(6). https://doi.org/10.1097/ta.0b013e318246efe5.

12. Ricci WM, Mamczak C, Tynan M, et al. Pelvic inlet and outlet radiographs redefined. J Bone Joint Surg 2010;92(10). https://doi.org/10.2106/JBJS.I.01580.

13. Graves ML, Routt MLC. Iliosacral screw placement: Are uniplanar changes realistic based on standard fluoroscopic imaging? J Trauma Inj Infect Crit Care 2011;71(1). https://doi.org/10.1097/TA.0b013e31821e842a.

14. Eastman JG, Chip Routt ML. Correlating preoperative imaging with intraoperative fluoroscopy in iliosacral screw placement. J Orthop Traumatol 2015;16(4). https://doi.org/10.1007/s10195-015-0363-x.

15. Weisz G, Houang M, Gollogly S. Re: Roussouly P, Gollogly S, Berthonnaud E, et al. Classification of

the normal variation in the sagittal alignment of the human lumbar spine and pelvis in the standing position. Spine 2005;30:346–53 [3] (multiple letters). Spine (Phila Pa 1976). 2005;30(13). doi:10.1097/01.brs.0000167527.42783.76.

16. Lee HD, Jeon CH, Won SH, et al. Global Sagittal Imbalance Due to Change in Pelvic Incidence after Traumatic Spinopelvic Dissociation. J Orthop Trauma 2017;31. https://doi.org/10.1097/BOT.0000000000000821.

17. Pekmezci M, Rotter P, Toogood P, et al. Reexamination of pelvic inlet and outlet images using 3-dimensional computed tomography reconstructions. J Orthop Trauma 2014;28(6). https://doi.org/10.1097/BOT.0000000000000018.

18. Conflitti JM, Graves ML, Chip Routt ML. Radiographic quantification and analysis of dysmorphic upper sacral osseous anatomy and associated iliosacral screw insertions. J Orthop Trauma 2010;24(10). https://doi.org/10.1097/BOT.0b013e3181dc50cd.

19. Scott WW, Magid D, Fishman EK, et al. Three-dimensional imaging of acetabular trauma. J Orthop Trauma 1987;1(3).

20. Keating TC, Bohl DD, Hamid KS. A Review of Fluoroscopic Image-Intensifier Artifacts and the Next Generation of Isocentric C-Arm Imaging. JBJS Rev 2018;6(12). https://doi.org/10.2106/JBJS.RVW.18.00013.

21. Kagan BD, Roberts MS, Haimes MA, et al. Intraoperative Comparative Femoral Rotation Imaging: Do not Overlook Parallax. J Orthop Trauma 2022;36(8). https://doi.org/10.1097/BOT.0000000000002347.

22. Williams THD, Syrett AG, Brammar TJ. W.S.B.-A fluoroscopy C-arm communication strategy. Injury 2009;40(8). https://doi.org/10.1016/j.injury.2008.10.011.

23. Yeo CH, Gordon R, Nusem I. Improving operating theatre communication between the orthopaedics surgeon and radiographer. ANZ J Surg 2014;84(5). https://doi.org/10.1111/ans.12482.

24. Burke JF, Anciano V, Novicoff WM, et al. Use of standardized language for c-arm fluoroscopy improves intraoperative communication and efficiency. J Am Acad Orthop Surg 2021;29(9):e458–64.

25. Gosselin MM, Dennis GS, Gary JL. The Utility of the Hyperinlet View in Posterior Fixation of Pelvic Ring Injuries. J Orthop Trauma 2022;36(5). https://doi.org/10.1097/BOT.0000000000002265.

26. Cunningham BA, Ficco RP, Swafford RE, et al. Modified iliac oblique-outlet view: A novel radiographic technique for antegrade anterior column screw placement. J Orthop Trauma 2016;30(9). https://doi.org/10.1097/BOT.0000000000000628.

27. Zhang L, Zhang W, Mullis B, et al. Percutaneous anterior column fixation for acetabulum fractures, does it have to be difficult? - The new axial pedicle

28. Quercetti N III, Horne B, DiPaolo Z, et al. Gun barrel view of the anterior pelvic ring for percutaneous anterior column or superior pubic ramus screw placement. Eur J Orthop Surg Traumatol 2017;27:695–704.

29. Guimarães JAM, Martin MP, da Silva FR, et al. The obturator oblique and iliac oblique/outlet views predict most accurately the adequate position of an anterior column acetabular screw. Int Orthop 2019;43(5). https://doi.org/10.1007/s00264-018-3989-5.

30. Norris BL, Hahn DH, Bosse MJ, et al. Intraoperative fluoroscopy to evaluate fracture reduction and hardware placement during acetabular surgery. J Orthop Trauma 1999;13(6):414–7.

31. Carmack DB, Moed BR, McCarroll K, et al. Accuracy of detecting screw penetration of the acetabulum with intraoperative fluoroscopy and computed tomography. J Bone Joint Surg 2001;83(9). https://doi.org/10.2106/00004623-200109000-00012.

32. Rashidifard C, Boudreau J, Revak T. Accuracy of Posterior Wall Acetabular Fracture Lag Screw Placement: Correlation between Intraoperative Fluoroscopy and Postoperative Computer Tomography. J Orthop Trauma 2020;34(12). https://doi.org/10.1097/BOT.0000000000001879.

33. Tosounidis TH, Giannoudis PV. Use of Inlet-Obturator Oblique View (Leeds View) for Placement of Posterior Wall Screws in Acetabular Fracture Surgery. J Orthop Trauma 2017;31(4). https://doi.org/10.1097/BOT.0000000000000724.

34. Wu X, Chen W, Zhang Q, et al. The study of plate-screw fixation in the posterior wall of acetabulum using computed tomography images. J Trauma Inj Infect Crit Care 2010;69(2). https://doi.org/10.1097/TA.0b013e3181ca05f6.

35. Swartz J, Vaidya R, Hudson I, et al. Effect of pelvic binder placement on OTA classification of pelvic ring injuries using computed tomography. Does it mask the injury? J Orthop Trauma 2016;30(6). https://doi.org/10.1097/BOT.0000000000000515.

36. Routt ML, Gary JL, Kellam JF, et al. Improved Intraoperative Fluoroscopy for Pelvic and Acetabular Surgery. J Orthop Trauma 2019;33. https://doi.org/10.1097/BOT.0000000000001403.

37. Sebaaly A, Jouffroy P, Moreau PE, et al. Intraoperative cone beam tomography and navigation for displaced acetabular fractures: A comparative study. J Orthop Trauma 2018;32. https://doi.org/10.1097/BOT.0000000000001324.

38. Ghisla S, Napoli F, Lehoczky G, et al. Posterior pelvic ring fractures: Intraoperative 3D-CT guided navigation for accurate positioning of sacro-iliac screws. J Orthop Traumatol: Surgery and Research 2018;104(7). https://doi.org/10.1016/j.otsr.2018.07.006.

39. Yang Z, Sheng B, Liu D, et al. Intraoperative CT-assisted sacroiliac screws fixation for the treatment of posterior pelvic ring injury: a comparative study with conventional intraoperative imaging. Sci Rep 2022;12(1). https://doi.org/10.1038/s41598-022-22706-y.

40. Verbeek J, Hermans E, van Vugt A, et al. Correct Positioning of Percutaneous Iliosacral Screws With Computer-Navigated Versus Fluoroscopically Guided Surgery in Traumatic Pelvic Ring Fractures. J Orthop Trauma 2016;30(6). https://doi.org/10.1097/00005131-201606000-00008.

41. Shaw J, Gary J, Ambrose C, et al. Multidimensional Pelvic Fluoroscopy: A New and Novel Technique for Assessing Safety and Accuracy of Percutaneous Iliosacral Screw Fixation. J Orthop Trauma 2020;34(11). https://doi.org/10.1097/BOT.0000000000001796.

Pediatrics

Neuromonitoring Changes in Spinal Deformity Surgery

Sterling Kramer, DO[a],*, Liz Ford, DO[b], Jed Walsh, DO[b]

KEYWORDS

- Neuromonitoring changes • Scoliosis • Cord injury • Motor evoked potential
- Somatosensory evoked potential

KEY POINTS

- Spinal cord injury is one of the most feared complications in spinal deformity surgery, with an incidence of major neurologic injury reported to range from 0.01% to 0.05%.
- By monitoring afferent and efferent pathways, spinal cord injury is detected early and potentially corrected before it becomes irreversible.
- Understanding the spinal cord anatomy, and the modes of monitoring for injury, helps the physician better understand the response to intraoperative signal changes.
- Having a well-defined, algorithmic protocol in place helps direct the response to intraoperative signal changes and avoid errors during these stressful moments.

INTRODUCTION

Injury to the spinal cord or exiting nerve roots is one of the most feared complications of spinal surgery.[1] The effects of intraoperative complications are devastating not only for the patient, but for the surgeon and all involved. The concept of the surgeon being the "second victim," and the hospital system being the "third victim" is well described in literature.[2,3] This refers to the psychological and financial impact these complications have on the surgeon and health care system and can have a ripple effect that goes well beyond those involved in the primary incident. Not all complications are created equally, and those in spine surgery have devastating, and potentially life-threatening repercussions. The presence of deformity, and associated variation in anatomic location of nerves and vessels augment the potential for these complications.[4] Patients and surgeons are aware of the potential complications of surgery, but little can prepare them for the psychological, mental, and emotional toll that one of these complications has. Fortunately, with improvements in neuromonitoring, the incidence of cord injury has significantly decreased.[5]

The cord depends on adequate perfusion to function, and is sensitive to mechanical changes. Thus injury to the cord can come either from direct trauma through errant screw placement, indirect trauma via hypoxic insult, or neuropraxic insult via stretch during correction.[6] The spinal cord consists of ascending sensory nerve fibers, and descending motor nerve fibers. During surgery, one or both are monitored to provide warning signs when there is injury to the cord, or an excessive amount of stress. Simultaneous multimodal monitoring provides nearly 100% sensitivity and specificity for injury,[7,8] so monitoring both is ideal. It is also best to have an experienced neuromonitoring technician in the room evaluating the feedback, because multiple studies have shown a direct relationship between experience and reliability in monitoring interpretations.[9,10] These same studies also show that there is an increased rate of postoperative neurologic deficit with less experience.

Even with an exceptional understanding of anatomy, and appropriate neuromonitoring, all surgeons experience intraoperative neuromonitoring changes in their career. The incidence of major neurologic injury is reported to range

---

[a] Campbell Clinic, Campbell Foundation, Suite 510, 1211 Union Avenue, Memphis, TN 38104, USA; [b] Inspira Health Network, 1505 West Sherman Avenue, Vineland, NJ 08360, USA
* Corresponding author.
E-mail address: skramerortho@gmail.com

Orthop Clin N Am 55 (2024) 89–99
https://doi.org/10.1016/j.ocl.2023.07.002

from 0.01% to 0.05%, with some centers reporting a monitoring change leading to an alert 13% of the time.[11,12] This is a stressful moment where all sources of injury must be considered to potentially reverse the cause and prevent long-term deficit. A surgeon's performance suffers under stress and time pressure,[6] and cortisol released during these moments can significantly impair memory retrieval.[13] It is best to avoid poor technique and acute memory loss during time critical moments in surgery, so having an established protocol printed and in the room as a visual aid for all to reference improves the efficiency of the team. Use of a checklist in crisis situations in the operating room resulted in a six-fold reduction in failure of adherence to critical steps in management.[6]

RELEVANT ANATOMY

The anatomy of the vertebral column is a complex circuit. The vertebral column is made up of osseous and neurovascular structures. Specifically of interest to this article, are anatomic structures that are at risk during deformity correction. The cervical, thoracic, and lumbar spine have variable pedicle morphology, which can pose a challenge during surgery. Specific to adolescent idiopathic scoliosis (AIS), Kuraishi and colleagues[14] found that pedicle morphology differs in patients with AIS, specifically in regards to the diameters. They noted the concave side of the deformity in patients with AIS was significantly narrower than the contralateral side, further suggesting that pedicle screw insertion for patients with AIS in the apex of the curve on the concave side should be avoided.

Kothe and colleagues[15] found that in the thoracic spine, the lateral cortex of the pedicle is significantly thinner than the medial cortex. Having a thicker medial cortex is protective when placing pedicle screws, because just medial to it lies the dura mater, and traversing nerve roots. In addition to the dangers medially to the pedicle, inferior to the pedicle also poses danger. The inferior wall of the pedicle is the roof of the neural foramen, with the exiting nerve root often abutting against it. Penetration through the medial or inferior wall of the pedicle has the potential for nerve injury and radicular pain from root irritation.[16]

One must also understand the crucial role of the spinal cord vascularity and associated structures in regard to cord perfusion. The spinal cord is sensitive to decreased perfusion, making monitoring blood pressure and limiting blood loss an important aspect of the procedure. The anterior two-thirds of the spinal cord receives its blood supply from one large anterior spinal artery, and the posterior one-third from paired posterior spinal arteries. These vessels anastomose via the arterial vasocorona, which wrap around the cord, supplying blood to the periphery and lateral aspects. There are large venous and arterial plexus surrounding the facet joints, that are prone to bleeding during facetectomies. Of note in the thoracic region, there is an area of decreased vascularity between T4 and T9, because it is the narrowest aspect of the spinal canal.[17] With most apical deformity in AIS located in these segments, perfusion is tenuous, and potential for injury increased.

There are ascending sensory and descending motor tracts that are important when specifically looking at neuromonitoring in deformity surgeries. More specifically, there are nine specific pathways that have distinct functions including movement, pain and temperature, position/fine touch, light touch, and short spinal connections (**Fig. 1**). A vascular insult or trauma may well affect these individual tracts in a unique way. For example, the dorsal columns that relay proprioception are dorsal-based tracts, and therefore more sensitive to blunt trauma. Most motor tracts are anterior, and are more sensitive to hypoperfusion from the blood supply.[17] Finally, the dysplastic nature of spinal deformity creates unique anatomy that is difficult to anticipate without appropriate preoperative imaging. Therefore, it is important to understand the relationships between anatomic structures and how to interpret changes in neuromonitoring while in the operating room.

TYPES OF NEUROMONITORING

There are many different ways of monitoring the spinal cord, each with their own nuances to consider. As noted earlier, the combined use of all types provides the best intraoperative prediction for postoperative neurodeficit.[7,8] The general concept is that an action potential is induced at one end of a nerve, and its latency and amplitude are evaluated at the other end after it has traveled the course of the nerve. The latency is a measure of time and distance, and the amplitude is a measure of power. When there is an increase in latency, or a decrease in amplitude higher than a certain threshold, this is a warning that the nerve is considered at risk for irreversible injury.

In somatosensory evoked potential (SSEP) monitoring, the action potential is propagated through the dorsal columns and dorsomedial tracts to the contralateral cerebral cortex. To

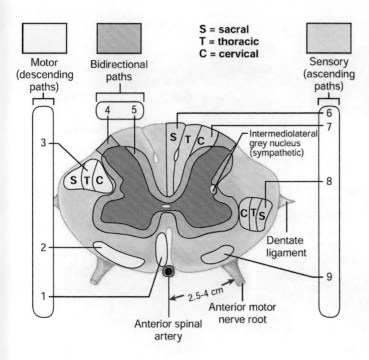

S = sacral
T = thoracic
C = cervical

Motor (descending paths)

Bidirectional paths

Sensory (ascending paths)

Intermediolateral grey nucleus (sympathetic)

Dentate ligament

2.5-4 cm

Anterior spinal artery

Anterior motor nerve root

Fig. 1. Cross-sectional anatomy of the spinal cord, showing the motor and sensory paths. These include the anterior corticospinal tract (1), vestibulospinal tract (2), lateral corticospinal (pyramidal) tract (3), dorsolateral fasciculus (4), fasciculus proprius (5), fasciculus gracilis (6), fasciculus cuneatus (7), lateral spinothalamic tract (8), and anterior spinothalamic tract (9). (With permission from "Frederick Azar, S. Terry Canale, James Beaty, Campbell's Operative Orthopaedics, 14th edition, v4. Philadelphia, PA, Elsevier Inc. 2021, chapter 37, pg 1643".)

do this, repetitive electrical stimulation of the peripheral nerves is instigated through epidural electrodes on the patient's skin at certain locations, and measured via subdermal electrodes on the scalp (Fig. 2). Different institutions have different thresholds, but generally an increase in latency by more than 10%, or a decrease in amplitude more than 50% initiates a warning to the surgeon of injury to these nerves.[18] SSEPs provide a good basic indicator of spinal cord function because they are continuously being evaluated; however, results need to be averaged over time to exclude background noise (Fig. 3). Because of this, they do not provide real-time feedback, and can take even up to 5 to 10 minutes to detect acute changes.[19] One study of 176 patients undergoing spinal surgery for deformity correction showed that SSEPs lagged MEPs by an average of 15 minutes when both were found to be positive.[20]

Motor evoked potentials (MEPs) allow selective and specific assessment of the functional integrity of descending motor pathways, from the motor cortex to the peripheral muscles.[18] These potentials are elicited by neurogenic stimulation at the spinal cord with epidural electrodes, or via myogenic stimulation through transcranial electrodes placed over the motor cortex on the scalp. Transcranial motor evoked potentials (TcMEPs) do not need to be averaged, and thus provide immediate response.

Typically a reduction in amplitude greater than 50% is a warning of injury. TcMEPs, however, are more sensitive to the effects of general anesthetics, which need to be considered before the start of surgery.

Another way of monitoring is via electromyography (EMG), which provides real-time recording from peripheral musculature.[19] Because EMG does not require stimulation, it can be continuously recording, and is most helpful with monitoring for injury to peripheral nerves, most often during pedicle screw placement. When a peripheral nerve is irritated, the associated innervated muscle shows spikes or bursts of activity on the EMG. One can also test each exiting nerve root selectively by electrically stimulating the pedicle screw at the associated level with increasing intensity. Because a well-placed screw is surrounded by cortical bone that insulates it, no activity should be seen at lower intensities. If neurotonic discharges are seen at less than 10 mA, one should suspect cortical breach of the screw, and should warrant further investigation.

The gold standard for ultimate assessment is the wake-up test, first described by Vauzelle and coworkers[21] in 1973, because all methods of cord monitoring have their inherent weaknesses. The surgeon should develop a routine that considers each individually, and uses multiple methods to avoid unnecessary surgical delay

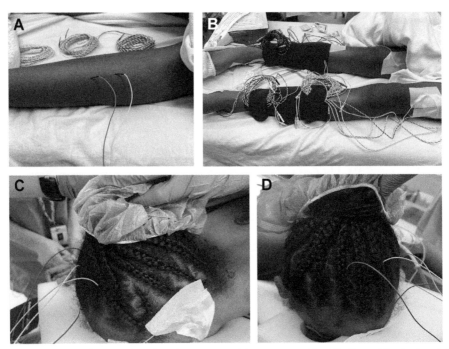

Fig. 2. Subdermal electrodes are placed in the upper and lower extremities (*A*, *B*), and in the head (*C*, *D*) for inducing and measuring action potentials in the motor and sensory tracts.

and risk by waking the patient to evaluate their neurologic status. SSEPs are easy to record, less affected by pharmacologic agents, and continuously record, but have delayed responses and may not provide warning until the injury is irreversible. There are reports of paralysis despite normal results of SSEPs.[22] TcMEPs provide instantaneous feedback, but

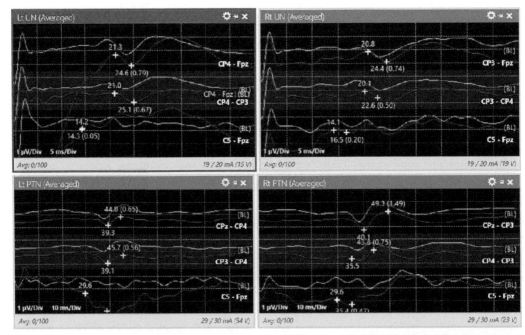

Fig. 3. Screen image of averaged SSEPs of bilateral upper and lower extremities. The *green lines* represent the baseline, and the *red lines* represent the current potentials.

are more sensitive to pharmacologic agents, cannot be constantly monitored, and are less accurate in kyphosis surgery.[12] Most institutions use a standard of continuous SSEPs and EMG, with TcMEPs performed at various checkpoints during the procedure, or when injury is suspected. Some routinely test pedicle screws with EMG after all are placed, removing the screw and palpating all cortices if the activity is seen lower than a certain threshold to confirm appropriate position of the screw. By combining all methods, one ensures the least likelihood of unexpected postoperative nerve deficit.

PERIOPERATIVE PATIENT SELECTION/RISK FACTORS FOR INTRAOPERATIVE NEURAL MONITORING LOSS AND INCREASE IN ELECTROPHYSIOLOGIC EVENTS

A successful surgery begins long before the patient enters the operating room. Appropriate patient selection and preoperative optimization is essential to minimize intraoperative risk. Although highly sensitive monitoring modalities can detect potentially reversible neurologic injury, there are medical comorbidities that can affect the reliability of one or both of these monitoring modalities, resulting in a statistically significant decrease in the likelihood of successful neurologic monitoring.

Vitale and coworkers reviewed 162 cases that demonstrated successful combined monitoring in 83% of spinal deformity surgeries.[12] Pelosi and colleagues[8] demonstrated similar results of 82%, success being defined by obtaining technically reproducible signals in sensory or motor stimulation under surgical conditions. Of the total patients unable to be monitored, risk factors included neuromuscular scoliosis, kyphosis, cerebral palsy, neuromuscular comorbidities, and anatomic comorbidities. Neuromuscular scoliosis, kyphosis, and cerebral palsy resulted in a statistically significant decrease in the ability of MEP monitoring to be obtained compared with idiopathic scoliosis. Cerebral palsy was also statistically less likely to have successful SSEP monitoring compared with idiopathic scoliosis. SSEP monitoring was trending to be less successful in neuromuscular scoliosis and kyphosis; however, statistical significance was not obtained. Neuromuscular comorbidities were less likely to be successfully monitored by MEP when compared with those patients without comorbidities. Even though these comorbidities decreased the likelihood to obtain one method of intraoperative neural monitoring (IONM), there was no difference found in the overall

success of combined IONM. More recent literature has corroborated these findings. Pastorelli and coworkers[23] demonstrated that IONM was reliable in patients with neuromuscular disease. However, the interpretation of IONM may be more challenging because the rate of false-positive results may be higher.[23] Hammett and colleagues[24] also stated that IONM is possible in neuromuscular patients but cautioned surgeons to take careful considerations when using IONM in this population.

In contrast, anatomic comorbidities, such as congenital anomalies, neoplasia, spondylolisthesis, and overgrowth, resulted in a decrease in the ability to monitor MEPs and SSEPs, and the overall success of the IONM.[6] Despite identifiable differences in success based on medical comorbidities, there is also a clear relationship with electrophysiologic changes and neurologic events.[12] Vitale and colleagues identified that surgeries involving spondylolisthesis, kyphosis, and cardiopulmonary comorbidities showed high rates of electrophysiologic events. Similarly, Feng and coworkers[20] identified kyphosis, procedures requiring osteotomies, and cobb angle corrections greater than 90° increased the likelihood of electrophysiologic events.

Besse and coworkers[25] investigated neuromonitoring in minimally invasive fusionless procedures for nonidiopathic scoliosis. They demonstrated an increase in loss of neurogenic mixed evoked potential monitoring (NMEP) in nonidiopathic patients undergoing surgery with large preoperative Cobb angles. Patients with central nervous system disease with elevated body mass index also demonstrated a statistically significant risk of NMEP signal loss.[25] They found no significant relationship between SSEP and NMEP loss with age, number of rods, upper instrumented vertebra, or lower instrumented vertebrae. However, the use of a traction table during surgery increased the risk of IONM loss.

Careful preoperative planning should take place in patients with medical comorbidities. MEP monitoring is less likely to be successfully obtained in neuromuscular scoliosis, kyphosis, cerebral palsy, and neuromuscular disease. SSEPs are difficult to obtain in cerebral palsy. During certain operations NMEP monitoring is affected by body mass index. Procedures involving corrections of large Cobb angles, kyphosis, spondylolisthesis, anatomic comorbidities, corrective osteotomies, and traction tables should be undertaken with increased caution because of the increase in risk of electrophysiologic events. The possibility of failure to obtain baseline neuromonitoring, increased risk of IONM loss, and decreases in the overall success of IONM in patients with comorbidities should be carefully considered by the operative surgeon.

SOURCES OF INJURY TO SPINAL CORD

Injury to the cord can come from several sources, but can ultimately be divided into direct trauma or secondary ischemia. Direct trauma is avoided by having a good knowledge of anatomy, appropriate operative technique, and sufficient intraoperative neuromonitoring. Secondary ischemia is avoided by preoperative patient optimization; intraoperative hemostasis; and maintaining vigilant watch over the patient's blood pressure, heart rate, and temperature. Although there is no definitive way of preventing all injuries, understanding the potential sources helps the surgeon have safe technique, and decrease the risk of complications.

Direct injury to the cord or exiting nerve root comes from errant screw placement, inadequate osteotomies, or traction during deformity correction. The anatomy of the thoracic pedicles in AIS is well described.[26,27] The pedicles of the apical and adjacent vertebrae are significantly shorter and narrower on the concave side, with an isthmus less than 4 mm in diameter in 62% of patients.[14] Furthermore, there are significant consequences of screw pullout, so choosing an appropriately sized screw is vital to construct stability. This anatomy, and the desire to place larger diameter pedicle screws make these pedicles more prone to screw breachment (Fig. 4), and potential nerve injury. Many surgeons rely on the concept of pedicle expansion; however, this decreases the overall pullout strength, and there is less expansion of the outer cortical diameter than the inner diameter.[28] Surgeon experience, and appropriate neuromonitoring help guide the choice of screw size and trajectory.

An extensive review of the Scoliosis Research Society morbidity and mortality database shows a 50% increase in complications, and more than double the amount of new neurologic deficit when osteotomies are performed.[1] Inadequate decompression can lead to ligament flavum involution and pressure on the cord, particularly on the convex side. Osteotomies also result in increased surgical time and blood loss, placing increased ischemic risk to the cord. A review of risks and costs associated with Ponte osteotomies from a different national database also showed no increased odds of neurologic complications, but did show 17.4% higher costs, 50% increase in readmissions, and 100% increase in reoperations within 90 days.[29]

Correction of the scoliosis also has a lengthening effect on the spine, with one study showing an average increase by 32.4 mm ± 10.8 mm.[30] The resulting lengthening of the spine can cause a traction neuropraxia resulting in postoperative neurodeficit (Fig. 5). This is also true with reduction of a spondylolisthesis. These patients are at a higher risk for cord injury,[12] with patients undergoing a reduction having a six-fold increased risk in new neurologic deficits.[1]

Secondary ischemia results from any factor that decreases the oxygenation of the cord. This is caused by hypotension, decreased hemoglobin, hypothermia, blood clots, intraoperative blood loss, or hematoma from vessel injury. Preoperative optimization is important because the rate of true electrophysical events is significantly higher in patients with cardiopulmonary comorbidities because of decreased oxygenation and perfusion.[12] During surgery, it is ideal to have background noises at an appropriate level, and the patient's vital signs displayed for all to see, so the whole team can be aware of any drastic changes. Hypotensive anesthesia during the surgical dissection can minimize blood loss, whereas maintaining Mean Arterial Pressures (MAPs) at 80 mm Hg ensures adequate cord perfusion during hardware placement and correction there is the highest risk of nerve injury.[19] One study showed that 20% of intraoperative signal changes improved by simply increasing the MAP to greater than 85 mm Hg.[30] Also, having an established standardized protocol in response to ischemic injury helps find the source, minimize the time to correction, and decrease the risk of irreversible injury.

USE OF A STANDARDIZED PROTOCOL

As mentioned previously, spinal surgery in scoliosis is stressful at baseline, with distorted anatomy and medically complicated patients. Hearing the neuromonitoring technician say that signals are diminished, or gone altogether increases the stress in the room and can easily result in poor surgeon performance, and difficulty with memory recall.[6,13] This is why the use of a standardized checklist is vital for management of these situations, because it puts everyone on the same page, gives everyone a role in finding and correcting the problem, and decreases time to correction by increasing efficiency. Although there are some published products that can be used,[6,31] there is not one that is better than another, and it is ideal that whichever you use is standardized to your institution. This limits variability for the supportive

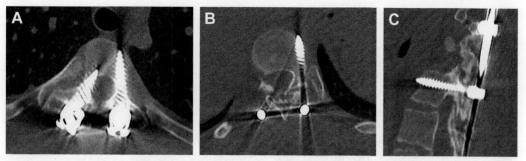

Fig. 4. Axial computed tomography showing a thoracic pedicle screw breaching the medial cortical wall (*A*) and lateral wall (*B*), and sagittal computed tomography of a thoracic pedicle screw breaching the anterior vertebral wall (*C*).

staff and improves the overall proficiency in the room. It should also be printed and visible in a known location. At our institution, the protocol is printed on a large poster board right next to the large monitor that displays the patient's vital signs (**Fig. 6**). It may even be beneficial to add its location, and assignments to the preoperative time out.

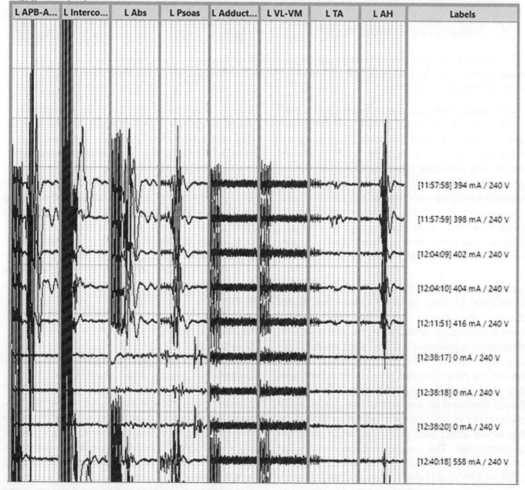

Fig. 5. Screenshot showing MEPs measured during the spinal correction in an AIS posterior spinal fusion. After final screw placement, all potentials were present and appropriate at 12:11. After correction of the spine to the rod, motors were lost in the left lower extremity at 12:38. Vitals and temperature were appropriate, so the correction was reversed, and the motors returned at 12:40.

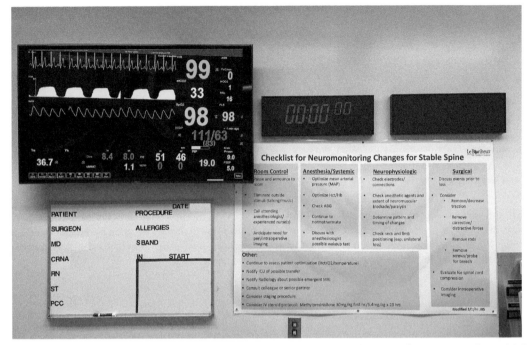

Fig. 6. This is an image of the wall in the operating rooms at our institution where spinal surgery is performed. It is always in view of the lead surgeon, and conveniently places the checklist next to the patient's vital signs, and the names of everyone in the room.

Whatever mode you use to organize the staff in the room, it should be simple and clear, and take into consideration the roles of the surgeon, anesthesiologist, and nursing staff. It should include the potential need for calling the assistance of senior staff, and the potential for advanced imaging with the patient anesthetized. The surgeon should also consider the timing in surgery where there were signal changes, because it is a clue to the cause. Next are general considerations that should be addressed.

General Considerations at all Times

Regardless of time at which there are signal changes, the surgeon should take control of the room by stopping; announcing the situation; and eliminating extraneous stimuli, such as music or side conversations.[6] The surgeon should verbally discuss any recent actions taken before the signal loss, and consider reversing them. Anesthesia should comment on any recent changes in use of pharmacologic agents, or changes in vital signs that would affect cord perfusion, and how it can be optimized. The neuromonitoring technician should specify which signals are affected (MEPs, SSEP, or EMG), and should consider any external causes, such as circuit discontinuity, electrode dislodgement, or electrical interference from external sources, such as cautery tools, magnetic devices, or warming blankets.

Signal Changes at Induction or Positioning

When there are signal changes before incision, the physician should check the leads, and consider transitioning to total intravenous anesthesia. The neuromonitoring technician should consider increasing baseline stimulation for SSEPs and anesthesia should consider decreasing propofol, which has a dose-dependent effect on MEP signals. Patient can be warmed, because hypothermia decreases signals, and as always, check patient positioning and vital signs. If signals do not return, consider aborting the case for a more extensive preoperative neurologic work-up.[19]

Signal Changes During or After Surgical Dissection

When signals change after exposure, it is likely caused by blood loss, anesthetics, or vital signs. Increase blood pressure to a MAP greater than 85 mm Hg[32] and warm the patient. Check an arterial blood gas and consider giving blood to maintain a hemoglobin greater than 7 mg/dL. Avoid boluses of propofol, considering a maximum dose of 150 μg/kg/min, because it is lipid-soluble and can accumulate with higher doses in heavier patients[33] and affect MEPs. If there is no improvement, consider a wakeup test, or aborting the case for further work-up.

Signal Changes During Screw Placement

When signals are lost during screw placement, the surgeon should still consider all things discussed previously; however, they must also consider the position of the screw and the concern that it is the offending agent. Simply evaluating the screw harmony, and its relationship to the other screws already placed can provide insight if it is malpositioned. A change in SSEPs could indicate a previously placed screw because of the delay from signal averaging, but spikes in EMG indicate acute irritation/injury to a nerve. The surgeon should promptly remove the screw and palpate the cortices of the pedicle, and consider individually testing the previous screws with EMG. The screw should be appropriately repositioned, or place hooks or sublaminar bands if an appropriate trajectory cannot be found.

Signal Changes with Osteotomies or Rod Placement/Correction

When there are signal changes during osteotomies, consider the degree of change and which pathway is affected. Motor pathways that are anterior may be more prone to perfusion, whereas sensory pathways that are posterior are more prone to direct insult. Evaluate the extent of the osteotomy to ensure there are no sharp edges that can impinge or irritate the cord, and ensure adequate hemostasis. If there are signal changes during rod placement and correction, immediately reverse the most recent action. If osteotomies were performed, make sure excess soft tissue and bone was removed. Once again, consider previously stated causes after the reversal to rule out any other potential cause. Consider a wake up test, and in situ fixation to allow further work-up if necessary.

Signal Changes During Closure or Postoperative

When there are signal changes during closure, particularly changes in SSEPs, consider it a delay in response and reverse the correction to see if it returns to baseline. Ensure the fluid you wash the wound out with is warm because the cord is sensitive to temperature change. If there were intraoperative changes at any point in time, consider admission to pediatric intensive care unit for a higher level of blood pressure monitoring and neuromuscular evaluation. If there are postoperative deficits with no intraoperative signal changes, consider drain output, intraoperative blood loss, and the need for advanced imaging.

SUMMARY

Although cord/nerve injury is a feared complication in scoliosis spine surgery, the overall complication rate is low, with incidence of major neurologic injury reported to range from 0.01% to 0.05%.[1,11,12] This is primarily because of better preoperative planning, and improvements in the ability to monitor the cord. Simultaneous monitoring of multiple pathways improves the detection of injury to nearly 100%.[7,8] Having an understanding of the different types of nerve monitoring and their individual strengths and weaknesses helps surgeons decide what is being injured and how to correct it. Also, having an established protocol in these situations maintains surgeon and staff composure, improves proficiency, and decreases the chances of the patient waking up with a nerve deficit.

CLINICS CARE POINTS

- Monitoring afferent and efferent pathways provides early detection of spinal cord injury, significantly decreasing incidence of irreversible cord damage.

- Use of an experienced neuromonitoring technician increases accuracy of monitoring, and decreases false-positive warnings.

- Having a well-defined, algorithmic protocol in place helps direct the response to intraoperative signal changes and avoid errors during these stressful moments.

- SSEPs lag behind because of averaging values, therefore monitoring sensory pathways alone can provide delayed warnings, theoretically increasing risk of irreversible injury.

- Decreasing thresholds for neuromonitoring alerts increases the sensitivity of cord injury, but decreases the specificity for true cord injury, resulting in false-positive alerts.

DISCLOSURES

None.

REFERENCES

1. Fu KMG, Smith JS, Polly DW, et al. Morbidity and mortality associated with spinal surgery in children: a review of the Scoliosis Research Society morbidity and mortality database. J Neurosurg Pediatr 2011; 7:37e41.

2. Wu AW. Medical error: the second victim. Br Med J 2000;320(7237).

3. Scott SD, Hirschinger LE, Cox KR, et al. The natural history of recovery for the healthcare provider "second victim" after adverse patient events. Qual Saf Health Care 2009;18(5):325–30.

4. Weiss HR, Goodall D. Rate of complications in scoliosis surgery: a systematic review of the Pub Med literature. Scoliosis 2008;3:9.

5. Charalampidis A, Jiang F, Wilson JRF, et al. The use of intraoperative neurophysiological monitoring in spine surgery. Global Spine J 2020;10(1 Suppl):104S–14S.

6. Vitale MG, Skaggs DL, Pace GI, et al. Best practices in intraoperative neuromonitoring in spine deformity surgery: development of an intraoperative checklist to optimize response. Spine Deform 2014;2(5):333–9.

7. Sutter M, Eggspuehler A, Muller A, et al. Multimodal intraoperative monitoring: an overview and proposal of methodology based on 1,017 cases. Eur Spine J 2007;16(suppl 2):S153e61.

8. Pelosi L, Lamb J, Grevitt M, et al. Combined monitoring of motor and somatosensory evoked potentials in orthopaedic spinal surgery. Clin Neurophysiol 2002; 113:1082–91.

9. Nuwer MR, Dawson EG, Carlson LG, et al. Somatosensory evoked potential spinal cord monitoring reduces neurologic deficits after scoliosis surgery: results of a large multicenter survey. Electroencephalogr Clin Neurophysiol 1995;96:6e11.

10. Stecker MM, Robertshaw J. Factors affecting reliability of interpretations of intraoperative evoked potentials. J Clin Monit Comput 2006;20:47e55.

11. Bridwell KH, Lenke LG, Baldus C, et al. Major intraoperative neurologic deficits in pediatric and adult spinal deformity patients. Incidence and etiology at one institution. Spine 1998;23:324–31.

12. Vitale MG, Moore DW, Matsumoto H, et al. Risk factors for spinal cord injury during surgery for spinal deformity. J Bone Joint Surg Am 2010;92(1):64–71.

13. Shields GS, Sazma MA, McCullough AM, et al. The effects of acute stress on episodic memory: a meta-analysis and integrative review. Psychol Bull 2017; 143:636–75.

14. Kuraishi S, Takahashi J, Hirabayashi H, et al. Pedicle morphology using computed tomography-based navigation system in adolescent idiopathic scoliosis. J Spinal Disord Tech 2013;26(1):22–8.

15. Kothe R, O'Holleran JD, Liu W, et al. Internal architecture of the thoracic pedicle: an anatomic study. Spine 1996;21(3):264–70.

16. Li G, Lv G, Passias P, et al. Complications associated with thoracic pedicle screws in spinal deformity. Eur Spine J 2010;19(9):1576–84.

17. Azar F, Terry Canale S, James B. 14th edition. Campbell's operative orthopaedics, v4. Philadelphia, PA: Elsevier Inc.; 2021. p. 1643. chapter 37.

18. Park JH, Hyun SJ. Intraoperative neurophysiological monitoring in spinal surgery. World J Clin Cases 2015;3(9):765–73.

19. Spitzer A, Patel R, Hasan S, et al, POSNA QSVI Committee. Absent baseline intraoperative neuromonitoring signals part I: adolescent idiopathic scoliosis: current concept review. Journal of the Pediatric Orthopaedic Society of North America 2022; 4(1). https://doi.org/10.55275/JPOSNA-2022-0018.

20. Feng B, Qiu G, Shen J, et al. Impact of multimodal intra-operative monitoring during surgery for spine deformity and potential risk factors for neurological monitoring changes. J Spinal Disord Tech 2012; 25(4):E108–14.

21. Vauzelle C, Stagnara P, Jouvinroux P. Functional monitoring of spinal cord activity during spinal surgery. Clin Orthop Relat Res 1973;93:173–8.

22. Ben-David B, Haller G, Taylor P. Anterior spinal fusion complicated by paraplegia. A case report of a false-negative somatosensory-evoked potential. Spine 1987;12:536–9.

23. Pastorelli F, Di Silvestre M, Vommaro F, et al. Intraoperative monitoring of somatosensory (SSEPs) and transcranial electric motor-evoked potentials (tce-MEPs) during surgical correction of neuromuscular scoliosis in patients with central or peripheral nervous system diseases. Eur Spine J 2015;24(Suppl 7):931–6.

24. Hammett TC, Boreham B, Quraishi NA, et al. Intraoperative spinal cord monitoring during the surgical correction of scoliosis due to cerebral palsy and other neuromuscular disorders. Eur Spine J 2013;22(Suppl 1):S38–41.

25. Besse M, Gaume M, Eisermann M, et al. Intraoperative neuromonitoring in non-idiopathic pediatric scoliosis operated with minimally fusionless procedure: a series of 290 patients. Arch Pediatr 2022;29(8):588–93.

26. Sato T, Nojiri H, Okuda T, et al. Three-dimensional morphological analysis of the thoracic pedicle and related radiographic factors in adolescent idiopathic scoliosis. BMC Musculoskelet Disord 2022; 23:847.

27. Demiroz S, Erdem S. Computed tomography-based morphometric analysis of thoracic pedicles: an analysis of 1512 pedicles and their correlation with sex, age, weight and height. Turk Neurosurg 2020;30(2):206–16.

28. Yazici M, Pekmezci M, Cil A, et al. The effect of pedicle expansion on pedicle morphology and biomechanical stability in the immature porcine spine. Spine 2006;31(22):E826–9.

29. Shaheen M, Koltsov JCB, Cohen SA, et al. Complication risks and costs associated with Ponte osteotomies in surgical treatment of adolescent idiopathic scoliosis: insights from a national database. Spine Deform 2022;10(6):1339–48.

30. Watanabe K, Hosogane N, Kawakami N, et al. Increase in spinal longitudinal length by correction surgery for adolescent idiopathic scoliosis. Eur Spine J 2012;21(10):1920–5.

31. Jain A, Khanna AJ, Hassanzadeh H. Management of intraoperative neuromonitoring signal loss. Semin Spine Surg 2015;27:229–32.

32. Yang J, Skaggs D, Chan P, et al. Raising mean arterial pressure alone restores 20% of intraoperative neuromonitoring losses. Spine 2018;43:890–4.

33. Cortínez LI, Fuente NDL, Oliveros A, et al. Performance of propofol target-controlled infusion models in the obese: pharmacokinetic and pharmacodynamic analysis. Anesth Analg 2014;119:302–10.

Shoulder and Elbow

Maximizing Implant Stability in the Face of Glenoid Bone Stock Deficiency

Austin F. Smith, MD[a], Mark A. Frankle, MD[a,b],
Kevin J. Cronin, MD[a,b],*

KEYWORDS

- Total shoulder arthroplasty • Reverse shoulder arthroplasty • Revision shoulder arthroplasty
- Glenoid bone loss • Glenoid wear • Shoulder arthroplasty • Shoulder

KEY POINTS

- Preoperative planning is essential to fully understand and account for glenoid bone loss.
- Options for primary anatomic total shoulder arthroplasty include eccentric reaming, bone grafting, or augmented glenoid components.
- Revision shoulder arthroplasty can lead to large glenoid defects requiring the use autograft or allograft, alternate center line, an augmented baseplate, or a combination of these techniques.
- Patient-specific or custom implants may provide an additional option for the treatment of severe glenoid bone loss though more research is needed.

INTRODUCTION

The incidence of shoulder arthroplasty continues to increase as indications for both anatomic and reverse shoulder arthroplasty expand to include primary osteoarthritis, inflammatory conditions, rotator cuff insufficiency, trauma, instability, and post-traumatic conditions. With these expanding indications, encountering glenoid bone loss in primary glenohumeral osteoarthritis, rotator cuff tear arthropathy (CTA), inflammatory arthritis, post-traumatic arthritis, or revision shoulder arthroplasty situations has become more commonplace.[1] With improved surgical techniques, advancement of both anatomic and reverse glenoid components, and the introduction of custom implants surgeons continue to tackle increasingly difficult cases of severe glenoid bone loss. To effectively and efficiently treat severe glenoid bone loss, surgeons must understand the common patterns of glenoid bone loss and the available reconstruction techniques including allograft, autograft, augmentation, and custom implants.

There are numerous classification systems to help better understand the common patterns of glenoid bone loss. In primary glenohumeral osteoarthritis, posterior wear is often encountered. Posterior glenoid bone loss can result in a decreased glenoid vault, medialization of the joint line, posterior humeral head subluxation, and loss of subchondral bone.[2] Neer first described the posterior humeral head subluxation and a sloped glenoid morphology in 1982.[3] Later, Walch provided a more detailed description of posterior glenoid bone loss in 1999.[4] This was expanded on by Iannotti in 2017 with the addition of B3 and C2 subtypes.[5] The Walch classification remains the most widely used classification system for primary posterior glenoid bone loss. It has been shown that 40-50% of patients with primary glenohumeral osteoarthritis have some form of posterior glenoid bone loss.[2,4]

[a] Florida Orthopaedic Institute, 13020 North Telecom Parkway, Temple Terrace, FL 33647, USA; [b] Department of Orthopaedic Surgery and Sports Medicine, University of South Florida, Florida Orthopaedic Institute, 13020 N. Telecom Parkway, Temple Terrace, FL 33647, USA
* Corresponding author.
E-mail address: kcronin@floridaortho.com
Twitter: @kevincroninmd (K.J.C.)

Orthop Clin N Am 55 (2024) 101–111
https://doi.org/10.1016/j.ocl.2023.05.011
0030-5898/24/© 2023 Elsevier Inc. All rights reserved.

In contrast, rotator cuff tear arthropathy has a distinctively different morphology of glenoid bone loss, predominately superior glenoid wear, that has been best described by the Favard Classification.[6] In Frankle's series of 216 glenoids, 37.5% of patients had some form of glenoid bone loss.[7]

There is a subset of patients with primary glenoid bone loss that do not meet the typical classification schema. Frankle defined these groups by glenoid morphology first by defining normal and abnormal glenoid morphology. Those with significant glenoid erosion were categorized by erosion type: posterior, superior, global, anterior.[7] It is postulated that different glenoid morphologies offer insight into the natural history of the muscular imbalance due to rotator cuff dysfunction. Neer established nutritional and biomechanical theories for classic cuff tear arthropathy and this may help describe patients classified as having abnormal superior erosion as well as those with abnormal global erosion. Still others have normal glenoid morphology with minimal joint degeneration. Therefore, it is important to evaluate the glenoid morphology as a means to understand the glenohumeral mechanics that are likely in place and may affect the durability of procedure performed and technique utilized.

Multiple classification systems have been suggested to account for bone loss in the revision scenario. These have been limited due to their reproducibility and ability to accurately quantify bone loss with prior implants in place.

PATIENT EVALUATION

There continues to be a significant debate on the most accurate and reliable imaging sequence to appropriately assess glenoid bone loss. Diagnosis of glenoid bone loss should begin with standard radiographic series including anteroposterior, Grashey, Scapular Y, and axillary views. It is vital to obtain reproducible and accurate radiographs on all patients with a concern for glenoid bone loss. The axillary view is particularly useful for determining Walch classification of bone loss however this has been shown to overestimate glenoid retroversion.[8] Posterior humeral head subluxation can also be appreciated on scapular Y and axillary two-dimensional (2D) imaging.[9] The true AP, or Grashey, view shows the geometric relationship of the humeral head to the glenoid to determine the registry of the humeral head in the glenoid. It should be noted that the widely accepted Walch classification was originally described validated based on radiographs only.

In cases of significant bone loss, a computed topography (CT) scan is useful for the assessment of the glenoid morphology and bone quality.[10–12] There has also been support for three-dimensional (3D) reconstruction to assess glenoid bone loss.[13–17] Frankle demonstrated that radiographic evaluation is adequate in cases of normal glenoid morphology, and that in cases with abnormal morphology 2D CT scan, and especially 3D CT scan reconstruction, led to higher reliability in diagnosis and preoperative planning.[7]

Finally, 3D pre-operative planning software has become more readily available and more widely utilized by surgeons to assess patients with advanced glenoid bone loss and deformity. This planning software provides automated measurements of glenoid morphology which have been shown to be both accurate and reliable compared to 2D imaging. These software programs allow for the virtual positioning of both anatomic and reverse glenoid components to optimize positioning and assess for version, inclination, and glenoid bone loss. Variation between measurements exists between each virtual planning implant system. Studies have shown that pre-operative planning predicts the need for an augmented glenoid component and influences intra-operative decision. Clinical studies have yet to demonstrate the benefit of these software applications.[2]

TREATMENT OPTIONS

In a patient with significant glenoid bone loss, the goals of surgery should be the restoration of function and pain relief utilizing an implant that provides adequate fixation and longevity. There are limits to both anatomic and reverse shoulder arthroplasty implant systems which must be considered.

BONE LOSS IN ANATOMIC TOTAL SHOULDER ARTHROPLASTY

In the setting of a patient otherwise indicated for anatomic total shoulder arthroplasty (aTSA), glenoid bone loss may be addressed by high-side reaming, bone grafting, or utilizing an augmented component. The goal of anatomic arthroplasty is near complete bone to implant backside contact. To accomplish this, the glenoid must be carefully reamed to accommodate the backside of the implant while being careful to preserve the subchondral bone plate. Limited reaming can lead to improper seating and early failure. On the contrary, over-reaming risks exposure of subchondral bone which provides inferior fixation. Additionally, posterior bone loss can lead to significant retroversion which must be, at least partially, corrected to aid in soft tissue balancing across the glenohumeral joint.

BONE GRAFTING

Though less commonly utilized due to increased failure rates, bone grafting remains an option in anatomic total shoulder arthroplasty with significant glenoid bone loss. Hill and Norris evaluated 17 patients at follow-up of 5.8 years treated with aTSA and bone grafting. Excellent and satisfactory result was seen in 3 and 6 patients, respectively. Of the remaining 8 patients there was graft failure in 3, glenoid loosening in 3, and instability in 2.[18] Scalise and Iannotti evaluated the conversion of failed aTSA to hemi with glenoid grafting with 3.2-year follow-up of 11 patients. There was graft subsidence seen in all patients with greater that 5 mm subsidence seen in 8 patients.[19]

ECCENTRIC REAMING

Eccentric reaming, or "high side reaming," to correct glenoid retroversion is an option to obtain adequate fixation of an anatomic glenoid component. Eccentric reaming has been shown to be successful in correcting 12-17 degrees of retroversion.[20,21] Gillespie demonstrated in a cadaveric study with simulated posterior bone loss of increasing increments of five degrees, that 50% of cases with 15 degrees of retroversion could not be corrected due to insufficient bone stock with eccentric reaming.[22] Iannotti demonstrated in a clinical study that patients with more than 18-20 degrees of retroversion cannot be corrected to zero degrees of version or patient-specific version without glenoid vault perforation when using a standard glenoid component.[23] This was confirmed in a computer simulation study by Nowak.[20] Ho followed 66 patients with a pegged glenoid component for 2-8 years and found osteolysis of the center peg in 20 cases (30%).[24] There was a fivefold increase of osteolysis around the glenoid center peg in patients that underwent aTSA with greater than 15 degrees of retroversion.

ANATOMIC AUGMENTED GLENOID

The use of an augmented glenoid component allows for the correction of greater defects and medialized glenoid bony erosion. Options include step-cut, half-wedge, or full-wedge augmented components. Multiple biomechanical studies have demonstrated comparable outcomes to standard implants. Short-to mid-term clinical studies have also shown promise. Wright and colleagues[25] found posterior glenoid components with 8 and 16 degrees of correction to have similar outcomes with no failures or revisions when compared to control at minimum 2-year follow-up. Another retrospective study of B2 and B3 glenoids treated with augmented anatomic implants showed favorable clinical and radiographic outcomes at 2-year follow-up.[26] The use of augmented glenoid components in aTSA may lead to favorable outcomes in a historically difficult patient population while providing the ability to restore glenohumeral anatomic relationships and preservation of normal biomechanical function. Long-term clinical studies are needed to confirm early data.

BONE LOSS IN PRIMARY REVERSE SHOULDER ARTHROPLASTY

In some scenarios, severe bone loss may result in the decision to use a reverse shoulder arthroplasty (RSA) implant due to insufficient glenoid bone stock and greater fixation strength with RSA baseplates. In patients without significantly abnormal glenoid morphology, centralized or eccentric reaming is sufficient to gain adequate baseplate fixation. Minzuno and Klein demonstrated that RSA is an effective treatment method for biconcave glenoids with significant glenoid bone loss.[27,28] McFarland showed RSA to be an effective treatment for patients with A2, B2, and C glenoids with 11 degrees of retroversion.[29] Forty-two patients were followed for an average of 36 months with an average ASES score of 73 and average elevation of 117 degrees. There was 1 case of glenoid failure and revision surgery.

BONE LOSS IN REVISION REVERSE SHOULDER ARTHROPLASTY

The number of primary RSA and aTSA performed per year increased substantially from 2012 to 2017 and is continuing to grow.[1] With this, the revision arthroplasty burden continues to increase. From 2012 to 2018 there were 61,615 revision shoulder arthroplasties performed in the United States, with 5,650 performed in 2012 and 14,300 performed in 2018 demonstrating a 153% increase. This is projected to increase to 37,329 in 2030.[1] (Fig. 1) In the revision shoulder arthroplasty setting, RSA is most commonly performed as it has

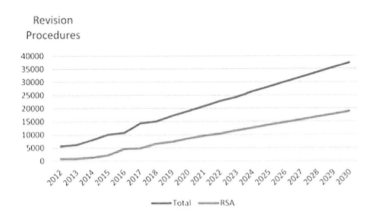

Fig. 1. Predicted increase in revision shoulder arthroplasty procedures from 2018 to 2030 in the United States. RSA, reverse shoulder arthroplasty.[1]

shown to be an effective treatment for failed aTSA,[30,31] failed hemi arthroplasty,[32] and failed RSA.[33] It is vital to develop effective strategies to treat these difficult cases which are typically associated with significant glenoid bone loss.

Multiple surgical techniques have been described to address severe glenoid bone loss including bone grafting, alternate center line, and base plate augmentation. Specialized design considerations have also been presented to assist with enhanced fixation.

TECHNIQUES FOR REVERSE SHOULDER ARTHROPLASTY WITH SIGNIFICANT BONE LOSS

Revision of failed arthroplasties may result in larger glenoid bone defects requiring structural grafting. It is important to first evaluate and understand the type of defect. Oftentimes, this is not possible pre-operatively due to metal artifact and inability to utilize pre-operative planning software in the revision situations. Currently, pre-operative planning in revision arthroplasty is available on some, but not all, commercial platforms. Antuna proposed a classification system to describe glenoid bone loss in revision shoulder arthroplasty. It is based on intraoperative findings and accounts for both the location (central, peripheral, combined) and severity (mild, moderate, severe) of the defect.[34] A modification was later proposed to describe the contained and uncontained defects.[35]

Typically, smaller peripheral defects can be managed without structural grafting while utilizing the remaining glenoid vault to achieve fixation. However, revision arthroplasty commonly leads to a central defect after removal of a previous baseplate. Often this can be a combined defect involving the central and peripheral glenoid rim.

BONE GRAFTING

Bone grafting has been shown to be an effective option in multiple studies.[28,36,37] In smaller central defects, crushed cancellous allograft may be adequate. In severe central and combined glenoid defects, structural graft, either allograft or autograft, may be preferred. In the revision setting, autologous bone graft may be used from the iliac crest. Alternatively, allograft femoral head allograft remains a viable option. Wagner evaluated 142 RSAs performed as a revision procedure with minimum 2-year follow-up.[38] Forty patients with bone grafting and 102 patients without bone grafting were compared. Of the 40 that underwent bone grafting, 14 (35%) utilized autograft from the iliac crest or humerus, 20 (50%) utilized allograft, and 6 (15%) utilized a combination of autograft and allograft. They found a 2 and 5-year revision-free survival of 88% and 76%, respectively, for those undergoing glenoid bone grafting. This was lower than that of patients who had not required glenoid bone grafting. There was no evidence of radiographic loosening in 92% and 88% of the shoulders at 2 and 5 years, respectively. Similarly, this was a higher rate of radiographic loosening then those who did not require bone grafting. Finally, the author's demonstrated significant pain relief, improvement in range of motion, and increased patient satisfaction in those undergoing glenoid reconstruction with allograft or autograft bone. Alternatively, Namdari followed 44 patients undergoing RSA with structural bone grafting including 7 revision cases. These authors found a 25% radiographic failure rate at a median of 8 months.[39] There have also been concerns regarding glenoid bone grafting including graft resorption and failure.[40]

The preferred surgical technique for bone grafting glenoid defects involves the preparation of the native glenoid to enhance the incorporation of the graft. The graft should be cut down and shaped to fit the defect on the back table. Once the graft is appropriately sized and shaped it should be secured to the native glenoid with multiple Kirschner wires outside of the area of planned glenoid reaming. One secured to the native glenoid, the central guidewire or pin can be placed followed by cannulated reaming of the native glenoid and the graft. Once the baseplate is appropriately seated, the peripheral Kirschner wires are removed (Fig. 2A-B). Fixation of the graft is achieved through compression as well as baseplate peripheral screws (Fig. 3A-C).

ALTERNATE CENTER LINE

In primary RSA, the central screw or post of the glenoid baseplate should match the native glenoid version and follow the anatomic center line. In the setting of severe glenoid bone loss this principle may lead to inadequate seating of the glenoid baseplate and early failure. To account for this, Frankle described the alternate center line. Scapula morphology (Fig. 4) involves 3 columns of bone: the coracoid base, the scapular spine, and the scapular pillar. The alternate center line captures the column of bone parallel to the scapular spine which is preserved in cases of severe glenoid bone loss (Fig. 5). Frankle evaluated the lengths of the standard center line and the alternate center line in normal and abnormal glenoids.[7] They found that in the normal glenoid the standard center line was 28.6 ± 4.1 mm and the alternative center line was 42.7 ± 19.1 mm; in the abnormal glenoid the standard center line was 19.6 ± 9.2 mm and the alternative center line was 34.9 ± 17 mm. It was further demonstrated that the anteversion required to achieve the alternative centerline compared to the standard center line was 9.2 degrees in the normal glenoid and 20.2 degrees in glenoids with posterior erosion. Colley evaluated 22 patients treated with alternative center line compared to a 3:1 matched cohort of 66 patients with baseplate placement along the anatomic center line.[41] At minimum 2-year follow-up the authors found similar outcomes for SST, ASES score, VAS pain score, SANE score, and active motion. No radiographic findings of baseplate failure were seen in either group. There were 2 cases of acromion fracture (9% vs 3%) in each cohort. In a comparative study by Klein, 143 shoulders were followed for two years. Fifty-six patients were treated with alternative center line for glenoid bone loss and 87 patients were treated with anatomic center line. There were no differences in ASES score at final follow-up.[28] The alternate center line is a technique that allows for adequate baseplate fixation in cases of severe glenoid bone loss in both revision and primary setting.

AUGMENTED GLENOID COMPONENTS

Augmented glenoid baseplates were first introduced to the United States in 2011 and have been used as an option for severe glenoid bone loss.[42] Virk demonstrated excellent clinical outcomes and no cases of aseptic loosening at an average follow-up of 40 months when evaluating 67 patients treated for osteoarthritis with RSA with an 8 degree posterior augmented baseplate.[43] Jones compared 41 patients treated with structural bone graft to 39 patients treated with an augmented baseplate and found similar outcomes in the reduction of pain, range of motion, and functional outcome scores with higher

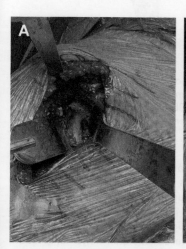
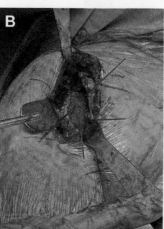

Fig. 2. (A) Right shoulder with deltopectoral approach showing large anterior glenoid bone defect. (B) Right shoulder with humeral head autograft utilized to fill the anterior glenoid bone defect. Three 2.0 mm Kirschner wires hold the autograft in place. The bone graft has been sculpted around the center guide wire for a cannulated reaming system. The guidewire has been placed into the alternate center line.

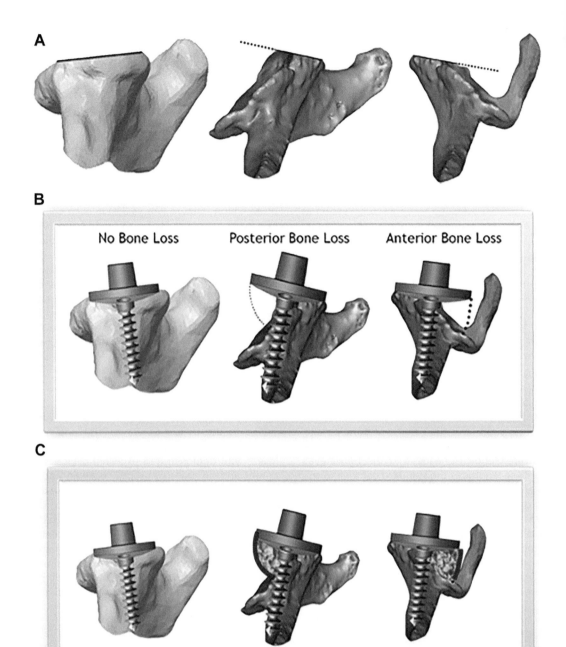

Fig. 3. (*A*) 3D glenoid model shoulder normal anatomy, posterior glenoid bone loss, and anterior glenoid bone loss. (*B*) 3D glenoid model showing baseplate positioning across the anatomic center line with no bone loss as well as an alternate center line with both posterior and anterior bone loss. (*C*) 3D glenoid model showing baseplate positioning across the anatomic center line with no bone loss as well as an alternate center line with both posterior and anterior bone loss with the addition of bone graft to fill the defect.

rates of complications and scapular notching in the patients undergoing structural bone graft.[42] Levin evaluated patients undergoing RSA in the setting of glenoid deformity and rotator cuff deficiency.[44] In this multicenter study 84 patients were treated with a standard baseplate design with a preoperative retroversion of 9 degrees, and 87 patients were treated with a baseplate with a wedge augmentation with a preoperative retroversion of 17 degrees. At >5 year follow-up they found significantly better postoperative abduction, forward flexion, and internal rotation also significantly higher in the augmented cohort (78 vs 65 and 81 vs 71, respectively). The rate of revision was similar in augmented and standard baseplate cohorts (0.7% and 3.0%, respectively).

Levine performed a systematic review comparing bone grafting to augmented baseplate and found no differences in clinical outcomes, complication rates or revision rates.[40] However, there was increased scapular notching and a higher rate of infection in the bone grafting group.

Augmented baseplates are an effective tool for the management of glenoid bone loss. However, these implants can be restrictive based on their design. Typically, options include fixed angle full or half wedge implants which are not always able to fully accommodate the glenoid defect. Pre-operative planning is vital to ensure appropriate seating of the augmented glenoid component.

DESIGN CONSIDERATIONS

Recent innovations in the glenosphere and baseplate design have focused on enhancing fixation in situations of significant glenoid bone loss. Nigro demonstrated that hooded glenoid implants provided multiple benefits in the revision setting.[45] In combination with the use of bone graft, these implants provide the ability to capture the bone graft while increasing the total interface area of the glenosphere therefore

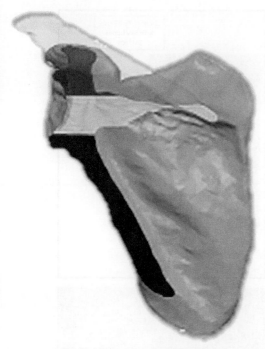

Fig. 4. Scapula morphology highlighting three distinct columns of bone: the coracoid base (red), the scapular spine (yellow), and the scapular pillar (blue).

in the augmented cohort. ASES scores were significantly higher in the augmented cohort versus the standard baseplate cohort (87 vs 76, respectively). Constant and SAS scores were

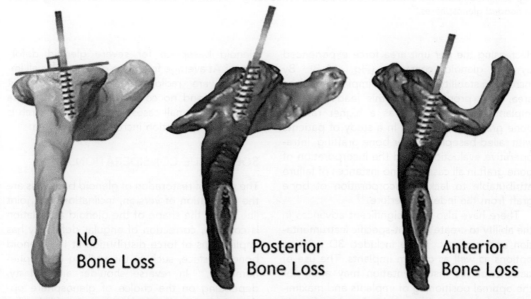

No Bone Loss

Posterior Bone Loss

Anterior Bone Loss

Fig. 5. 3D glenoid model showing baseplate positioning down the anatomic center line as well as the alternate center line with posterior and anterior glenoid bone loss. The baseplate captures the column of bone parellel to the scapular spine which remains preserved in cases of severe glenoid bone loss.

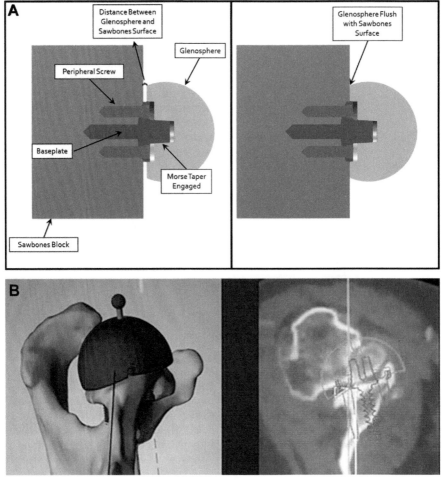

Fig. 6. (A) Biomechanical considerations in the use of hooded glenospheres. (B) 3D glenoid model showing the use of hooded glenospheres.[45]

decreasing the per unit area force experienced by the glenoid construct (Fig. 6A-B). By increasing stability and glenoid implant interface area, it is proposed that this leads to high implant stability as well as a higher rate of bone graft incorporation. In a study of patients with failed baseplates after bone grafting, intraoperative evaluation found the incorporation of bone graft in all cases and no instances of failure attributable to lack of incorporation of bone graft from the index procedure.[33]

There have also been significant advances in the ability to create patient-specific instrumentation and implants. These included 3D printing options as well as custom implants. The use of patient-specific instrumentation may allow for the optimal positioning of implants and maximization of the glenoid bone-implant interface in cases of severe glenoid bone loss. Murthi reported results of 11 shoulders after custom

glenoid baseplate for severe glenoid deformity.[46] At average follow-up of 30 months all implants were radiographically stable without loosening and no complications. Overall, data is limited to small cases and further research is needed as innovation increases in this area.

SOFT TISSUE CONSIDERATIONS

The goals of restoration of glenoid bone loss are the restoration of version, inclination, and joint line. Since the shape of the glenoid articulation is concave, correction of angular deformity has implications of force distribution at the glenoid bone interface, such as the rocking horse phenomenon.[47] In reverse shoulder arthroplasty, depending on the choice of glenosphere options include a hemisphere or two-thirds of a sphere. In this scenario, the degree of correction of version and inclination is less important since a convex surface has a greater ability to neutralize these asymmetric forces. The greater the sphericity, the less angular deformity becomes an issue.

However, the soft tissue envelope becomes a consideration in terms of the relationship of the humerus to the glenoid. In osteoarthritis, it is largely assumed and observed that the muscles are healthy, and if the contracted capsule is resected, restoring the joint line and native shape of the humerus and glenoid allows for idealized kinematics to occur.

When RSA is used for primary osteoarthritis, an attempt to optimize these same kinematics is a goal by restoring the humeral-glenoid relationship which allows the restoration of tension and direction of muscle forces. However, in other pathologies (ie CTA, failed rotator cuff surgery, inflammatory arthritis, and so forth), the soft tissues are of greater concern. An attempt to restore the soft tissues to the premorbid length can lead to irrecoverable stiffness or increased joint reactive forces which can lead to implant/bone interface failure.

An alternative approach is to plan to optimize the component fixation of the glenoid that would include maximizing the bony contact with the center screw or peg with less emphasis on baseplate glenoid contact area.[48] Next, the selection of the glenosphere can be adjusted to tension the diseased soft tissues if they are patulent. Larger spheres will provide tension while a smaller sphere can be used in situations of contracted soft tissues. When planning for a bone loss case in primary osteoarthritis, the bone loss is a reflection of soft tissues and resecting a diseased capsule helps significantly. However, in other pathologies such as cuff tear arthropathy or inflammatory arthritis, be prepared to adjust your reconstruction to accommodate the appropriate pathology.

SUMMARY

Glenoid bone loss represents a wide spectrum of disease from various etiologies with multiple treatment options. Stereotypical forms of glenoid bone loss that meet typical classification schema have been well studied and treatment algorithms have been proposed. As glenoid bone loss becomes more significant, careful evaluation must be undertaken. Patients with significant glenoid bone loss require advanced techniques and/or implants to adequately treat their pathology. Further, the rate of patients requiring revision shoulder arthroplasty is increasing and this group represents a unique

and difficult challenge in terms of glenoid bone loss. Patients in the revision setting will often have combined defects that require the consideration of bone grafting, use of the alternative centerline, and specialized implants. It is important to have an appropriate preoperative plan approaching these difficult cases as they may require nonstandard equipment and materials, and the incidence of these cases is likely to increase.

CLINICS CARE POINTS

- Always obtain appropriate pre-operative imaging including radiographs and CT scans. Utilization of pre-operative planning software can provide substantial benefit to understanding glenoid bone loss and enhance surgical planning.

- Options for bone loss in primary anatomic total shoulder arthroplasty include bone grafting, eccentric reaming, or augmented glenoid components.

- Options for bone loss in primary or revision reverse shoulder arthroplasty include bone grafting, augmented glenoid components, or use of the alternative center line.

- Additionally, various intraoperative techniques can enhance the fixation of the glenoid component and improve long-term outcomes.

- Custom, or patient-specific, implants may provide an additional option for patients with significant glenoid bone loss though long-term data are lacking.

DISCLOSURE STATEMENT

Dr A.F. Smith has nothing to disclose. Dr K.J. Cronin receives consulting fees from Enovis Surgical. Dr M.A. Frankle receives consulting and royalty fees from Enovis Surgical.

REFERENCES

1. Best MJ, Aziz KT, Wilckens JH, et al. Increasing incidence of primary reverse and anatomic total shoulder arthroplasty in the United States. J Shoulder Elbow Surg 2021;30(5):1159–66.
2. Cronin KJ, Kirsch JM, Gates S, et al. Three-dimensional measures of posterior bone loss and retroversion in Walch B2 glenoids predict the need for an augmented anatomic glenoid component. J Shoulder Elbow Surg 2021;30(10):2386–92.

3. Neer CS 2nd, Watson KC, Stanton FJ. Recent experience in total shoulder replacement. J Bone Joint Surg Am 1982;64(3):319–37.

4. Walch G, Badet R, Boulahia A, et al. Morphologic study of the glenoid in primary glenohumeral osteoarthritis. J Arthroplasty 1999;14(6):756–60.

5. Iannotti JP, Jun BJ, Patterson TE, et al. Quantitative measurement of osseous pathology in advanced glenohumeral osteoarthritis. J Bone Joint Surg Am 2017;99(17):1460–8.

6. Levigne C, Boileau P, Favard L, et al. Scapular notching in reverse shoulder arthroplasty. J Shoulder Elbow Surg 2008;17(6):925–35.

7. Frankle MA, Teramoto A, Luo ZP, et al. Glenoid morphology in reverse shoulder arthroplasty: classification and surgical implications. J Shoulder Elbow Surg 2009;18(6):874–85.

8. Nyffeler RW, Jost B, Pfirrmann CW, et al. Measurement of glenoid version: conventional radiographs versus computed tomography scans. J Shoulder Elbow Surg 2003;12(5):493–6.

9. Khan AZ, Hendy BA, Kohan EM, et al. Scapular Y: the forgotten radiograph in glenohumeral arthritis—novel measurement of posterior humeral head subluxation on scapular Y radiographs. Semin Arthroplasty: JSES. 2022;32(3):490–6.

10. Couteau B, Mansat P, Mansat M, et al. In vivo characterization of glenoid with use of computed tomography. J Shoulder Elbow Surg 2001;10(2):116–22.

11. Friedman RJ, Hawthorne KB, Genez BM. The use of computerized tomography in the measurement of glenoid version. J Bone Joint Surg Am 1992;74(7):1032–7.

12. Mullaji AB, Beddow FH, Lamb GH. CT measurement of glenoid erosion in arthritis. J Bone Joint Surg Br 1994;76(3):384–8.

13. Budge MD, Lewis GS, Schaefer E, et al. Comparison of standard two-dimensional and three-dimensional corrected glenoid version measurements. J Shoulder Elbow Surg 2011;20(4):577–83.

14. Ganapathi A, McCarron JA, Chen X, et al. Predicting normal glenoid version from the pathologic scapula: a comparison of 4 methods in 2- and 3-dimensional models. J Shoulder Elbow Surg 2011;20(2):234–44.

15. Kwon YW, Powell KA, Yum JK, et al. Use of three-dimensional computed tomography for the analysis of the glenoid anatomy. J Shoulder Elbow Surg 2005;14(1):85–90.

16. Scalise JJ, Bryan J, Polster J, et al. Quantitative analysis of glenoid bone loss in osteoarthritis using three-dimensional computed tomography scans. J Shoulder Elbow Surg 2008;17(2):328–35.

17. Verstraeten TR, Deschepper E, Jacxsens M, et al. Operative guidelines for the reconstruction of the native glenoid plane: an anatomic three-dimensional computed tomography-scan reconstruction study. J Shoulder Elbow Surg 2012;21(11):1565–72.

18. Hill JM, Norris TR. Long-term results of total shoulder arthroplasty following bone-grafting of the glenoid. J Bone Joint Surg Am 2001;83(6):877–83.

19. Scalise JJ, Iannotti JP. Bone grafting severe glenoid defects in revision shoulder arthroplasty. Clin Orthop Relat Res 2008;466(1):139–45.

20. Nowak DD, Bahu MJ, Gardner TR, et al. Simulation of surgical glenoid resurfacing using three-dimensional computed tomography of the arthritic glenohumeral joint: the amount of glenoid retroversion that can be corrected. J Shoulder Elbow Surg 2009;18(5):680–8.

21. Ting FS, Poon PC. Perforation tolerance of glenoid implants to abnormal glenoid retroversion, anteversion, and medialization. J Shoulder Elbow Surg 2013;22(2):188–96.

22. Gillespie R, Lyons R, Lazarus M. Eccentric reaming in total shoulder arthroplasty: a cadaveric study. Orthopedics 2009;32(1):21.

23. Iannotti JP, Greeson C, Downing D, et al. Effect of glenoid deformity on glenoid component placement in primary shoulder arthroplasty. J Shoulder Elbow Surg 2012;21(1):48–55.

24. Ho JC, Sabesan VJ, Iannotti JP. Glenoid component retroversion is associated with osteolysis. J Bone Joint Surg Am 2013;95(12):e82.

25. Wright TW, Grey SG, Roche CP, et al. Preliminary results of a posterior augmented glenoid compared to an all polyethylene standard glenoid in anatomic total shoulder arthroplasty. Bull Hosp Jt Dis 2015;73(Suppl 1):S79–85.

26. Ho JC, Amini MH, Entezari V, et al. Clinical and radiographic outcomes of a posteriorly augmented glenoid component in anatomic total shoulder arthroplasty for primary osteoarthritis with posterior glenoid bone loss. J Bone Joint Surg Am 2018;100(22):1934–48.

27. Mizuno N, Denard PJ, Raiss P, et al. Reverse total shoulder arthroplasty for primary glenohumeral osteoarthritis in patients with a biconcave glenoid. J Bone Joint Surg Am 2013;95(14):1297–304.

28. Klein SM, Dunning P, Mulieri P, et al. Effects of acquired glenoid bone defects on surgical technique and clinical outcomes in reverse shoulder arthroplasty. J Bone Joint Surg Am 2010;92(5):1144–54.

29. McFarland EG, Huri G, Hyun YS, et al. Reverse total shoulder arthroplasty without bone-grafting for severe glenoid bone loss in patients with osteoarthritis and intact rotator cuff. J Bone Joint Surg Am 2016;98(21):1801–7.

30. Walker M, Willis MP, Brooks JP, et al. The use of the reverse shoulder arthroplasty for treatment of failed total shoulder arthroplasty. J Shoulder Elbow Surg 2012;21(4):514–22.

31. Black EM, Roberts SM, Siegel E, et al. Reverse shoulder arthroplasty as salvage for failed prior

arthroplasty in patients 65 years of age or younger. J Shoulder Elbow Surg 2014;23(7):1036–42.

32. Levy J, Frankle M, Mighell M, et al. The use of the reverse shoulder prosthesis for the treatment of failed hemiarthroplasty for proximal humeral fracture. J Bone Joint Surg Am 2007;89(2):292–300.

33. Holcomb JO, Cuff D, Petersen SA, et al. Revision reverse shoulder arthroplasty for glenoid baseplate failure after primary reverse shoulder arthroplasty. J Shoulder Elbow Surg 2009;18(5):717–23.

34. Antuna SA, Sperling JW, Cofield RH, et al. Glenoid revision surgery after total shoulder arthroplasty. J Shoulder Elbow Surg 2001;10(3):217–24.

35. Malhas A, Rashid A, Copas D, et al. Glenoid bone loss in primary and revision shoulder arthroplasty. Shoulder Elbow 2016;8(4):229–40.

36. Neyton L, Walch G, Nove-Josserand L, et al. Glenoid corticocancellous bone grafting after glenoid component removal in the treatment of glenoid loosening. J Shoulder Elbow Surg 2006;15(2):173–9.

37. Melis B, Bonnevialle N, Neyton L, et al. Glenoid loosening and failure in anatomical total shoulder arthroplasty: is revision with a reverse shoulder arthroplasty a reliable option? J Shoulder Elbow Surg 2012;21(3):342–9.

38. Wagner E, Houdek MT, Griffith T, et al. Glenoid bone-grafting in revision to a reverse total shoulder arthroplasty. J Bone Joint Surg Am 2015;97(20):1653–60.

39. Ho JC, Thakar O, Chan WW, et al. Early radiographic failure of reverse total shoulder arthroplasty with structural bone graft for glenoid bone loss. J Shoulder Elbow Surg 2020;29(3):550–60.

40. Lanham NS, Peterson JR, Ahmed R, et al. Comparison of glenoid bone grafting versus augmented glenoid baseplates in reverse shoulder arthroplasty: a systematic review, J Shoulder Elbow Surg, 2022, S1058-2746(22)00326-3. Online head of print.

41. Colley R, Polisetty TS, Levy JC. Mid-term outcomes of reverse shoulder arthroplasty using the alternative center line for glenoid baseplate fixation: a case-controlled study. J Shoulder Elbow Surg 2021;30(2):298–305.

42. Jones RB, Wright TW, Roche CP. Bone grafting the glenoid versus use of augmented glenoid baseplates with reverse shoulder arthroplasty. Bull Hosp Jt Dis 2015;73(Suppl 1):S129–35.

43. Virk M, Yip M, Liuzza L, et al. Clinical and radiographic outcomes with a posteriorly augmented glenoid for Walch B2, B3, and C glenoids in reverse total shoulder arthroplasty. J Shoulder Elbow Surg 2020;29(5):e196–204.

44. Levin JM, Bokshan S, Roche CP, et al. Reverse shoulder arthroplasty with and without baseplate wedge augmentation in the setting of glenoid deformity and rotator cuff deficiency-a multicenter investigation. J Shoulder Elbow Surg 2022;31(12):2488–96.

45. Nigro PT, Gutierrez S, Frankle MA. Improving glenoid-side load sharing in a virtual reverse shoulder arthroplasty model. J Shoulder Elbow Surg 2013;22(7):954–62.

46. Bodendorfer BM, Loughran GJ, Looney AM, et al. Short-term outcomes of reverse shoulder arthroplasty using a custom baseplate for severe glenoid deficiency. J Shoulder Elbow Surg 2021;30(5):1060–7.

47. Franklin JL, Barrett WP, Jackins SE, et al. Glenoid loosening in total shoulder arthroplasty. Association with rotator cuff deficiency. J Arthroplasty 1988;3(1):39–46.

48. Formaini NT, Everding NG, Levy JC, et al. The effect of glenoid bone loss on reverse shoulder arthroplasty baseplate fixation. J Shoulder Elbow Surg 2015;24(11):e312–9.

Hand and Wrist

The Pitfalls of Difficult Distal Radius Fractures and Provisional Reduction

Jared A. Bell, MD[a], Nicholas F. James, MD[a,*],
Benjamin M. Mauck, MD[b], James H. Calandruccio, MD[b],
William J. Weller, MD[b]

KEYWORDS

- Distal radius • Distal radius fracture • Wrist fracture • Wrist fracture treatment
- Surgical techniques • Open reduction internal fixation • Provisional reduction

KEY POINTS

- Fractures of the distal radius can be challenging to treat and careful planning is required.
- Many different operative techniques are available to assist in provisional reduction and fracture fixation.
- Appropriate surgical approach, provisional reduction, and type of fixation play critical roles in treatment success.

INTRODUCTION

Incidence and Epidemiology

Distal radius fractures are commonly encountered injuries, comprising a sixth of all emergency department visits for fractures in the United States.[1] In elderly individuals, distal radius fractures are only secondary to hip fractures, with an incidence of 643,000 per year.[2,3] They have a bimodal distribution that involves high-energy trauma in younger, higher-demand populations and low-energy, often ground-level falls, in an elderly osteoporotic population.[4] The most frequent mechanism is a fall on an outstretched, pronated wrist with forces traveling from the hand through the distal radius, resulting in a dorsally and radially displaced fracture pattern.[5] Sporting activities and motor vehicle accidents account for a large proportion of these injuries in the young adult population. Despite the high incidence of distal radius fractures, debate remains over the methods of treatment

and the techniques involved, which is likely due to the lack of large, prospective randomized control trials on the topic.[6]

While operative treatment of distal radius fractures can be relatively straight forward, there are many factors that significantly increase the intra-operative complexity of obtaining a provisional reduction and stable fixation. Poor bone quality, significant bone loss, unstable fracture patterns, or highly comminuted injuries are some factors that increase the difficulty of operative treatment. This article will provide options that can be used to obtain satisfactory reduction of displaced distal radius fractures.

Operative Fixation

Historically, surgical treatment was less common and included limited percutaneous fixation in combination with immobilization. With the advent of the volar locking plate, open reduction and internal fixation techniques have increased in

[a] Department of Orthopedic Surgery, University of Florida Health Jacksonville, 655 8th Street West, Jacksonville, FL 32209, USA; [b] Campbell Clinic Department of Orthopedic Surgery, University of Tennessee Health Science Center, 7887 Wolf River Boulevard, Germantown, TN 38138, USA
* Corresponding author.
E-mail address: nicholas.james@jax.ufl.edu

Orthop Clin N Am 55 (2024) 113–122
https://doi.org/10.1016/j.ocl.2023.05.012

popularity due to more stable fixation allowing earlier range of motion.[7–10] Volar locking plate fixation is now the most common form of surgical fixation for distal radius fractures and offers a significant advantage over previous non-locking implant designs, particularly in osteoporotic bone.[4,11] The majority of displaced distal radius fractures are dorsally angulated and would theoretically be amenable to a buttress construct on the dorsal aspect of the distal radius. However, little soft-tissue coverage, typical dorsal comminution, decreased tolerance of dorsal scars, and the prominence of hardware leading to tendon irritation have all led to the rise of volar plate fixation.[12] Early removal of hardware did not necessarily preclude extensor tendon tenosynovitis or attritional rupture; however, newer dorsal implant designs have shown a decreased rate of these complications.[13–15] There are instances when a dorsal approach may be preferred, such as where there is a need for the direct observation of the articular surface or improved stability against dorsal collapse, and these should not be discounted.[16] A volar approach, although not without its own disadvantages, avoids the aforementioned issues and often provides a less comminuted cortex for fracture reduction, increased distance between the flexor tendons and the implant, better tolerated scars, and a lower chance of disturbing the blood supply of the radius.[17] The fixed-angle and polyaxial locking volar plate designs provide stable fixation even in instances of metadiaphyseal comminution by transferring forces from the distal fragments to the intact radial shaft, allowing for versatility of use with many different fracture types.[18] This article focuses on intra-operative techniques of provisional reduction and fracture fixation with many, but not all, of the solutions geared toward locked volar plating. While volar locking plate fixation is the most common method, it is important to consider other options for difficult distal radius fractures such as dorsal plating, percutaneous pinning, fragment-specific fixation, dorsal-spanning fixation, and external fixation, or a combination thereof.

Classification

Multiple classification systems exist for distal radius fractures. Useful classification systems should have a high degree of intraobserver and interobserver reliability to provide reproducible diagnostic, treatment, and prognostic value. Because of the significant variability of distal radius fracture morphologies and lack of high-quality evidence to direct treatment, current classification systems for these fractures have limited utility and tend to have high interobserver and intraobserver variability. Additionally, this has only been found to slightly improve with the use of computed tomography scans, which is not a standard practice for most distal radius fractures.[19] Instead, different classification systems historically tended to identify important characteristics of distal radius fracture patterns. In 1814 Colles first described dorsally angulated and displaced extra-articular distal radius fractures.[20] This is still the most common fracture pattern today and has since been renamed a "Colles" fracture. Several other eponyms have followed such as the Barton, Smith, die-punch, and Chauffer's fracture.[21] The development of the roentgenograph (circa 1895) led to the earliest attempts at classification systems, such as the Nissen-Lie system, in the 1930s,[22] and this was expanded by Gartland and Werley in 1951 and Lidstrom in 1959 to include fracture lines, degree and direction of displacement, and radiocarpal articular involvement.[23,24] Several other classification systems followed; the Frykman (1967), Fernandez (2001), Universal (1993), and the AO classification (1986) are the most common classification systems in use today.[25–28] The AO classification is the most frequently used and remains the most comprehensive system, utilizing 27 categories.[19] It was adopted by the Orthopedic Trauma Association in 2007, simplified to 9 categories, and renamed the "AO/OTA Classification of Fractures and Dislocations."[29] This modified version was an attempt to improve intraobserver and interobserver reliability. It has 3 types (extra-articular, partially articular, and complete articular), and each type has 3 groups based on fracture patterns, propagation, and comminution.[30] There is still significant debate among practitioners regarding which classification system best guides clinical treatment. Despite the shortcomings of the current classification systems, it is important to clearly characterize distal radius fractures prior to surgical treatment to guide approach, fixation type, and expected outcomes. Computed tomography can be useful for pre-operative planning when it is difficult to characterize the fracture pattern, especially articular congruity, and will help to prevent intra-operative pitfalls.[31]

SURGICAL PRINCIPLES
Bony and Ligamentous Anatomy

Before discussing possible surgical pitfalls, it is important to understand the typical fracture morphology and functional anatomy of the distal radius. The distal radius is composed of three different articulating surfaces: the scaphoid facet, the lunate facet, and the sigmoid notch. The scaphoid and lunate facets make up the distal aspect of the radius and articulate with their aptly named and respective carpal bones. The facets can be distinguished by a central ridge on the distal radius in line with the space between the scaphoid and lunate. The distal radius extends radially to form the radial styloid and radioscaphoid articulation. The distal radioulnar joint (DRUJ) is composed of the sigmoid notch, located on the ulnar aspect of the distal radius and often perpendicular to the radiocarpal joint line, and the distal ulna. The sigmoid notch has a radius of curvature about 4 to 7 mm larger than the ulnar head, which leads to dorsal translation in pronation and volar translation in supination.[32] Both intrinsic and extrinsic ligaments serve to stabilize the wrist articulations and translate forces to the radiocarpal joint. The most relevant intrinsic ligaments for wrist stabilization are the scapholunate and lunotriquetral interosseous ligaments as they maintain the proximal carpal row in smooth articulation with the distal radius. The primary extrinsic stabilizing ligaments of the radiocarpal joint include the radioscaphocapitate, radiolunotriquetral (long radiolunate ligament), radioscapholunate (short radiolunate ligament), and the dorsal radiotriquetral ligaments. The triangular fibrocartilage complex (TFCC) is composed of the articular disc, the meniscus homolog, the superficial and deep dorsal and volar radioulnar ligaments, and the ulnar collateral ligament which provides stability to the DRUJ.[33]

Three-Column Model

The three-column model was first described by Rikli and Regazzoni and is useful to consider when treating comminuted fractures.[34] The distal radius can be divided into three separate columns: medial (ulnar), intermediate, and lateral (radial) (Fig. 1).

The radial column includes the radial styloid and the scaphoid facet, which act to directly resist radial translation of the carpus. The radial column also provides appropriate radial height to allow for equal distribution of forces along the radiocarpal joint. It is the origin for the radioscaphocapitate and radial collateral ligaments that act to resist ulnar translation and provide stability to the carpus.[35] Importantly, the brachioradialis inserts on the radial styloid and acts as a deforming force in certain distal radius fractures, leading to radial shift, loss of radial height, and inclination.[36]

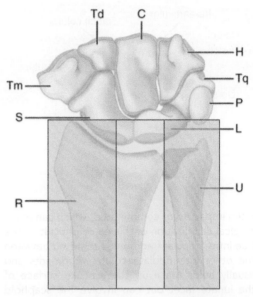

Fig. 1. Three column model: Blue - lateral/radial column, Green - intermediate column, Orange - medial/ulnar column. C, Capitate; H, hamate; L, lunate; P, pisiform; R, radius; S, scaphoid; Td, trapezoid; Tm, trapezium; Tq, triquetrum; U, ulna. (*Adapted from* Cannon, DL. Wrist Disorders. In Azar FM, Beaty JH (eds.). Campbell's Operative Orthopaedics, 13th edition, Philadelphia, Elsevier, 2021, pp. 3478.)

The intermediate column is the centerpiece of the model and acts to connect and direct forces from the columns to the shaft of the radius.[34,35,37] The intermediate column contains the sigmoid notch and the lunate facet, which can be further subdivided into key characteristic fracture fragments found in complex intra-articular distal radius fractures: the volar rim, dorsal ulnar corner, dorsal wall, and free intra-articular fragment (Fig. 2). The volar rim, or "critical corner" fragment, shares a portion of both the lunate facet and the sigmoid notch and is the attachment site of the radioscapholunate and volar distal radioulnar ligament. Inadequate fixation of this fragment can lead to volar carpal and DRUJ instability because of the strong ligamentous attachments. Malreduction can compromise the articular surface of both the radiocarpal joint and the DRUJ, leading to decreased motion and future degenerative complications.[36] The dorsal ulnar corner is the other fragment that makes up the sigmoid notch as well as the anchor for the dorsal radioulnar ligament and, therefore, similarly affects the DRUJ stability and kinematics required for pronation and supination. The dorsal wall is the attachment site for the dorsal radiocarpal ligament and helps to prevent dorsal carpal subluxation. It is

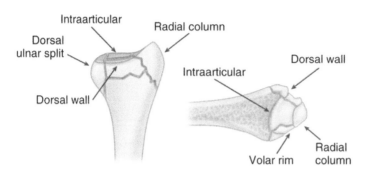

Fig. 2. Illustration of the subdivision of the intermediate column. (*Adapted from* Edward A. Perez. Fractures of the Shoulder, Arm and Forearm. In Azar FM, Beaty JH (eds.). Campbell's Operative Orthopaedics, 13th edition, Philadelphia, Elsevier, 2021, pp. 3005.)

often impacted or comminuted, which can make surgical stabilization of this piece difficult.[38] The free intra-articular fragment is centered between the other intermediate column fragments and usually helps make up the articular surface of the lunate facet but can involve the scaphoid facet. It is frequently impacted and may require tamping to restore the articular surface.

The ulnar column is composed of the distal ulna and the TFCC. It is instrumental in facilitating pronation-supination of the forearm and stabilization of the DRUJ. The ulnar column is generally treated after the fixation of the radial and intermediate columns if the DRUJ remains unstable, otherwise studies have shown no improvement in outcome with ulnar styloid fixation if the radius is anatomically reduced.[39]

Goals of Surgical Treatment

The goal of distal radius fracture treatment is to restore anatomic alignment as well as possible to achieve pain-free wrist and forearm motion, return to pre-injury activities, and decrease the likelihood of developing future complications. Restoration of anatomic alignment is ideal and always the initial goal, but this is not always possible. Intra-operative radiographic criteria for acceptable alignment includes:[40–42]

1. Radial inclination > 15°
2. Tilt between 10° dorsal tilt and 20° volar tilt
3. Radial shortening less than 2 mm
4. Radiocarpal intra-articular step-off or gap less than 2 mm
5. Sigmoid notch incongruity less than 2 mm
6. Ulnar variance less than 5 mm

CHALLENGES AND SURGICAL TECHNIQUES

Radial Shift or Loss of Radial Inclination

The radial inclination of the distal radius is measured on a posteroanterior radiograph from the intersection of one line perpendicular

to the long axis of the radial shaft and one line drawn from the distal tip of the radial styloid to the ulnar corner of the lunate fossa. A normal radial inclination is $22 \pm 3°$.[43,44] Radial shift is the radial translation of the distal radius fracture fragment and can be best appreciated on posteroanterior radiographs. It actually represents ulnar translation of the more proximal radial shaft. The brachioradialis insertion onto the radial styloid may translate deforming forces, causing both radial shift and loss of radial inclination of the distal fragment.[39] Efforts to correct this deformity for plate fixation can be a source of frustration because the radial styloid fragment can be relatively small and difficult to gain enough purchase to counteract the pull of the brachioradialis. In situations when a percutaneous Kirschner wire (K-wire) placed diagonally through the radial styloid tip to the intact ulnar cortex of the radial shaft is insufficient, we recommend considering a brachioradialis tenotomy. This can be performed routinely through a volar approach without meaningful functional consequences to strength or range of motion.[45–47] The brachioradialis tendon transected approximately 5 cm proximal to its insertion may be sutured to the volar capsule and the pronator quadratus reattached for plate coverage. After the brachioradialis tenotomy, axial traction and an ulnar-directed force can restore the radial inclination and reduce the radial shift. A point-to-point clamp also can be used with a tine on the radial aspect of the distal fragment and the other on the ulnar aspect of the shaft. A percutaneous K-wire is placed diagonally from the styloid to the intact shaft component prior to plate fixation. Additionally, a carefully placed Bennett retractor along the ulnar cortex of the proximal radial metaphysis can assist with the reduction of radial shift. Care must be taken to not do this for long periods or too aggressively because this can lead to median nerve neurapraxia. Placing two provisional K wires in the K-wire holes on the shaft part of the plate can also assist in maintaining the reduction of the translation deformity once adequate reduction is achieved. Last, the plate can be placed first on the distal articular block and fixated and then reduced to the shaft. This technique takes significant familiarity with plate placement and distal radius bone morphology to execute successfully; there is some guesswork in how to place the plate on the distal articular block to adequately restore radial inclination.

Loss of Radial Height

The distal radius radial height is measured on a posteroanterior radiograph as the distance between two lines perpendicular to the axis of the radial shaft, one in line with the tip of the radial styloid and the other drawn at the ulnar aspect of the lesser sigmoid notch articular surface. A normal radial height is about 14 ± 1 mm in adults. Greater than 3 mm of shortening meets the criteria for operative fixation.[48–50] Failure to restore radial height can result in loss of tendinous mechanical advantage and incongruency of the DRUJ. This can lead to loss of strength, impingement of the TFCC, and increased potential for ulnar head subluxation, leading to painful restriction of motion and ultimately degenerative arthritis.[51,52] The natural tension from the flexor and extensor tendons spanning the radiocarpal joint acts as a deforming force to reduce the radial length. Generally, the use of a

percutaneous axial K-wire at the styloid can provide adequate provisional fixation; however, in difficult distal radius fractures, this is not always possible. There are several other options for assisting with the provisional restoration of radial height such as placing an intra-operative finger-trap on the thumb or index finger, a dorsal-spanning wrist plate, or external fixator. These techniques rely on ligamentotaxis to restore the anatomy for successful reduction, and care should be taken to not over-distract and direct these forces through the radial column. Over-distraction of the carpus has been associated with extrinsic extensor tendon tightness limiting composite fist and may increase rates of complex regional pain syndrome (CRPS).[53,54] Volar plates with an oblong hole in the plate also can be used to restore height. This is accomplished by fixing the distal fragment to the plate and placing a cortical screw into the distal aspect of the oblong hole. Prior to tightening the shaft screw, axial traction is applied to the hand, which will move the plate distally, and the screw can be tightened within the proximal aspect of the oblong hole. An alternative is to use a point-to-point clamp, with one tine in the head of the loosened shaft screw and the other on the proximal aspect of the plate. As the clamp is compressed, it will shift the plate distally and the shaft screw can be tightened in the proximal aspect of the oblong hole, or a second screw can be placed in a different hole (**Fig. 3**).

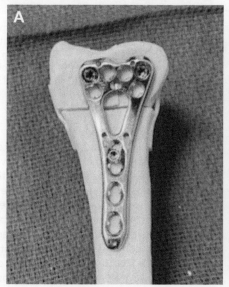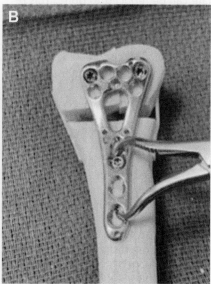

Fig. 3. (A) Example of fixing the distal fragment to the plate and placing a cortical screw into the distal aspect of the oblong hole prior to tightening the shaft screw. (B) Using a point-to-point clamp with one tine in the head of the loosened shaft screw and the other tine on the proximal aspect of the plate. As the clamp is compressed, the plate shifts distally and the shaft screw can be tightened in the proximal aspect of the oblong hole.

Loss of Volar Tilt

The volar tilt of the distal radius is measured on a lateral radiograph from the intersection of a line drawn along the axis of the radial shaft and a line perpendicular to a line connecting the volar and dorsal rims of the distal radius. The normal volar tilt is 11 ± 5°.[55] There is an inverse relationship between the volar tilt angle and the maximum joint reaction force that highly correlates with clinical outcomes.[56,57] Generally, the volar tilt can be restored manually with distal traction, volar flexion, and ulnar deviation of the hand and possibly provisionally held by percutaneous K-wire fixation. If direct manipulation does not fully correct the volar tilt, the plate can be leveraged, in a kickstand technique, to achieve further volar tilt.[58] For this technique the proximal aspect of the plate is intentionally lifted off of the shaft. To keep the proximal aspect of the plate off the bone, a short 10- to 12-mm screw can be placed into the proximal locking hole to act as a kickstand if needed (Fig. 4). A towel bump placed posterior to the radiocarpal joint on the hand table also is helpful. The plate is then fixed to the distal fragment. If difficulty is encountered drawing the distal fragment to bone, a cortical screw placed within a distal locking hole can compress the plate to bone or a lobster claw instrument can be used. This can be switched out for a peg or locking screws after the remaining distal holes are filled. The previously placed locking screw in the proximal shaft is removed, and the plate can be reduced to bone. This results in a "kick-stand" effect and increasing the volar tilt. This technique can be effective in the setting of dorsal comminution.[59]

Comminuted Intra-articular Fragments with Depression

A technique that can be effective in the setting of intra-articular fragments and dorsal comminution is a modified intrafocal pinning technique. Kapandji originally described an intrafocal pinning technique in 1987 that involved placing pins through the dorsal aspect of the fracture site and levering the distal fragment back into place to restore the volar tilt.[60] This is mostly effective for extra-articular fractures. The modified technique involves fixing a volar plate to the radial shaft without placing the distal screws. Then, a 2-mm K-wire is inserted dorsally through the fracture site and used to tamp any depressed fragments and restore the articular surface. Next, multiple dorsal subchondral wires are placed to provide fixation to the reduced articular surface and then leveraged

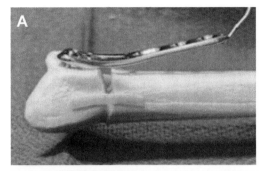

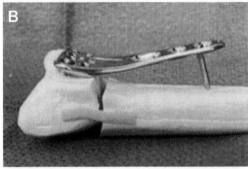

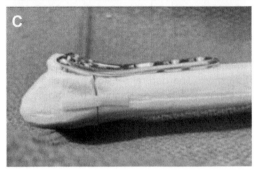

Fig. 4. (A) Image of the plate sitting off of the radial shaft proximally in this example with a dental pick. (B) Kickstand technique using a 10 to 12 mm locking screw to keep proximal aspect of the plate elevated. (C) Subsequent reduction with the proximal portion of the plate reduced to the radial shaft.

simultaneously to restore the volar tilt. Finally, the distal screws are placed to hold the reduced fracture in place, and the wires are removed.[61] If the metaphyseal void is small after elevating any depressed fragments and there is sufficient subchondral support of the articular surface, bone grafts or substitutes are not required because this will consolidate with time.[62,63] Larger voids, as seen with some die-punch fragments, may benefit from a structural augmentation such as cancellous allograft or calcium phosphate. Although autograft remains the gold standard for local bone defects, it is often not necessary for the healing of distal radius fracture and is associated with donor site morbidity and complications.[64,65] When direct fracture fixation is not possible, the indirect techniques previously discussed should be considered to restore anatomic alignment or a combination of direct and indirect techniques. The extended flexor carpi radialis (FCR) approach can be used for exposure of very distal fractures and allow for the intrafocal reduction of the joint surface against the proximal row.[66]

Volar Rim Fracture

The volar rim fragment is part of the lunate facet and sigmoid notch and is usually either dorsiflexed or volarly displaced.[55] Without anatomic reduction and stabilization, the carpus will subluxate volarly because of the strong ligament attachments to the volar rim. A volar buttress construct is necessary to ensure stabilization and to prevent later displacement.[36] The volar lunate facet fragment usually is a larger, triangular fragment and can be sufficiently buttressed with a conventional volar locked plate placed proximal to the watershed line. Occasionally, the volar rim fragment is comminuted, and a separate small and rectangular piece is found distal to the watershed line.[67] Fixation of this fragment cannot be achieved with a volar locking construct in isolation because it would require placement distal to the watershed line with plate prominence at the volar lip and high risk of

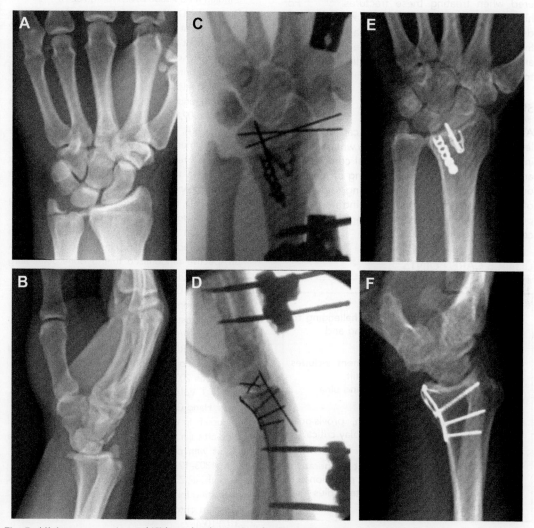

Fig. 5. (A) Anteroposterior and (B) lateral radiographs of a distal radius volar rim fragment with a concomitant ulnar styloid fracture. (C) Anteroposterior and (D) lateral fluoroscopic images of fracture-specific volar rim fixation using a buttress and hook plate. External fixation and supplemental Kirschner wires were utilized to stabilize the scapholunate and radiocarpal alignment. (E) Anteroposterior and (F) lateral post-operative radiographs with interval removal of the Kirschner wires and external fixator.

attritional tendon rupture unless it is later removed.[36] Instead, an additional construct is required; many options have been suggested and available. Different fixation options have been successfully used and include hook plates, bent K-wires, headless screws, wire loops, hook plate extensions, pin plates, and rim plates.[68–72] We recommend a fragment-specific implant such as a hook plate or bent K-wires (**Fig. 5**). K-wires are introduced volarly through the fragment, into the dorsal cortex, and bent to lay over the volar radius with enough length to lay under the volar plate. Reports of adequate exposure of the volar lunate facet have been reported with the extended FCR approach, but a volar-ulnar approach may be useful and can be considered when treating these fractures.[66,72,73] For highly comminuted fractures that cannot be directly fixed, a dorsal spanning plate or external fixator can be used to restore the overall anatomic alignment by utilizing ligamentotaxis to gain an indirect reduction.

SUMMARY

A complex fracture of the radius can be a challenging surgical problem especially when multiple intra-articular fragments or cortical comminution are present. Detailed understanding of the anatomy, thorough preoperative planning, knowledge of available treatment options, and intra-operative provisional reduction techniques are key to successful management.

CLINICS CARE POINTS

- Distal radius fractures can be challenging to treat and require careful planning and consideration
- Restoration of anatomic alignment includes the correction of radial height, tilt, inclination, articular congruity, and ulnar variance
- Appropriate surgical approach, provisional reduction, and type of fixation play critical roles in treatment success
- There are many different operative techniques available to assist in provisional reduction prior to definitive distal radius fracture fixation

DISCLOSURE

The authors have nothing to disclose.

REFERENCES

1. Ilyas AM, Jupiter JB. Distal radius fractures–classification of treatment and indications for surgery. Orthop Clin North America 2007;38(2):167–73, v.
2. Chung KC, Spilson SV. The frequency and epidemiology of hand and forearm fractures in the United States. J Hand Surg Am 2001;26(5):908–15.
3. Larsen CF, Lauritsen J. Epidemiology of acute wrist trauma. Int J Epidemiol 1993;22(5):911–6.
4. He JJ, Blazar P. Management of high-energy distal radius injuries. Curr Rev Musculoskelet Med 2019; 12(3):379–85.
5. Shaw R, Mandal A, Mukherjee KS, et al. An evaluation of operative management of displaced volar Barton's fractures using volar locking plate. J Indian Med Assoc 2012;110(11):782–4.
6. Downing ND, Karantana A. A revolution in the management of fractures of the distal radius? J Bone Joint Surg Br 2008;90(10):1271–5.
7. Abramo A, Kopylov P, Geijer M, et al. Open reduction and internal fixation compared to closed reduction and external fixation in distal radial fractures: a randomized study of 50 patients. Acta Orthop 2009;80(4):478–85.
8. Karantana A, Downing ND, Forward DP, et al. Surgical treatment of distal radial fractures with a volar locking plate versus conventional percutaneous methods: a randomized controlled trial. J Bone Joint Surg Am 2013;95(19):1737–44.
9. Rozental TD, Blazar PE, Franko OI, et al. Functional outcomes for unstable distal radial fractures treated with open reduction and internal fixation or closed reduction and percutaneous fixation. A prospective randomized trial. J Bone Joint Surg Am 2009;91(8):1837–46.
10. Koenig KM, Davis GC, Grove MR, et al. Is early internal fixation preferred to cast treatment for well-reduced unstable distal radial fractures? J Bone Joint Surg Am 2009;91(9):2086–93.
11. Larson AN, Rizzo M. Locking plate technology and its applications in upper extremity fracture care. Hand Clin 2007;23(2):269–78, vii.
12. Orbay J. Volar plate fixation of distal radius fractures. Hand Clin 2005;21(3):347–54.
13. Fitoussi F, Ip WY, Chow SP. Treatment of displaced intra-articular fractures of the distal end of the radius with plates. J Bone Joint Surg Am 1997; 79(9):1303–12.
14. Kamath AF, Zurakowski D, Day CS. Low-profile dorsal plating for dorsally angulated distal radius fractures: an outcomes study. J Hand Surg Am 2006; 31(7):1061–7.
15. Simic PM, Robison J, Gardner MJ, et al. Treatment of distal radius fractures with a low-profile dorsal plating system: an outcomes assessment. J Hand Surg Am 2006;31(3):382–6.

16. Lutsky K, Boyer M, Goldfarb C. Dorsal locked plate fixation of distal radius fractures. J Hand Surg Am 2013;38(7):1414–22.

17. Orbay JL, Touhami A. Current concepts in volar fixed-angle fixation of unstable distal radius fractures. Clin Orthop Relat Res 2006;445:58–67.

18. Schneppendahl J, Windolf J, Kaufmann RA. Distal radius fractures: current concepts. J Hand Surg Am 2012;37(8):1718–25.

19. Kleinlugtenbelt YV, Groen SR, Ham SJ, et al. Classification systems for distal radius fractures. Acta Orthop 2017;88(6):681–7.

20. Colles A. Historical paper on the fracture of the carpal extremity of the radius (1814). Injury 1970;2(1): 48–50.

21. Mauck BM, Swigler CW. Evidence-based review of distal radius fractures. Orthop Clin North Am 2018; 49(2):211–22.

22. Nissen-lie HS. Fracture radii "typical". Nord Med 1939;1:293–303.

23. Gartland JJ, Werley CW. Evaluation of healed Colles' fractures. J Bone Joint Surg Am 1951;33-A(4):895–907.

24. Lidstrom A. Fractures of the distal end of the radius. A clinical and statistical study of end results. Acta Orthop Scand Suppl 1959;41:1–118.

25. Frykman G. Fracture of the distal radius including sequelae–shoulder-hand-finger syndrome, disturbance in the distal radio-ulnar joint and impairment of nerve function. A clinical and experimental study. Acta Orthop Scand 1967;(Suppl 108):3+. https://doi.org/10.3109/ort.1967.38.suppl-108.01.

26. Fernandez DL, Geissler WB. Treatment of displaced articular fractures of the radius. J Hand Surg Am 1991;16(3):375–84.

27. Cooney WP. Fractures of the distal radius. A modern treatment-based classification. Orthop Clin North Am 1993;24(2):211–6.

28. Muller ME, Nazarian S, Koch P. Classification AO des fractures. 1st edition. Berlin: Springer-Verlag; 1987. Les os longs.

29. Marsh JL, Slongo TF, Agel J, et al. Fracture and dislocation classification compendium - 2007: Orthopaedic Trauma Association classification, database and outcomes committee. J Orthop Trauma 2007;21(10 Suppl):S1–133.

30. Jayakumar P, Teunis T, Giménez BB, et al. AO distal radius fracture classification: global perspective on observer agreement. J Wrist Surg 2017;6(1):46–53.

31. Cole RJ, Bindra RR, Evanoff BA, et al. Radiographic evaluation of osseous displacement following intraarticular fractures of the distal radius: reliability of plain radiography versus computed tomography. J Hand Surg Am 1997;22(5):792–800.

32. Ekenstam F, Hagert CG. Anatomical studies on the geometry and stability of the distal radio ulnar joint. Scand J Plast Reconstr Surg 1985;19(1):17–25.

33. Palmer AK, Werner FW. The triangular fibrocartilage complex of the wrist–anatomy and function. J Hand Surg Am 1981;6(2):153–62.

34. Rikli DA, Regazzoni P. Fractures of the distal end of the radius treated by internal fixation and early function. A preliminary report of 20 cases. J Bone Joint Surg Br 1996;78(4):588–92.

35. Rikli DA, Honigmann P, Babst R, et al. Intra-articular pressure measurement in the radioulnocarpal joint using a novel sensor: in vitro and in vivo results. J Hand Surg Am 2007;32(1):67–75.

36. Kennedy SA, Hanel DP. Complex distal radius fractures. Orthop Clin North Am 2013;44(1):81–92.

37. Rikli DA, Regazzoni P, Babst R. [Management of complex distal radius fractures]. Zentralbl Chir 2003;128(12):1008–13.

38. Rhee PC, Medoff RJ, Shin AY. Complex distal radius fractures: an anatomic algorithm for surgical management. J Am Acad Orthop Surg 2017;25(2): 77–88.

39. Koh S, Andersen CR, Buford WL, et al. Anatomy of the distal brachioradialis and its potential relationship to distal radius fracture. J Hand Surg Am 2006;31(1):2–8.

40. Nana AD, Joshi A, Lichtman DM. Plating of the distal radius. J Am Acad Orthop Surg 2005;13(3): 159–71.

41. Graham TJ. Surgical correction of malunited fractures of the distal radius. J Am Acad Orthop Surg 1997;5(5):270–81.

42. Altissimi M, Antenucci R, Fiacca C, et al. Long-term results of conservative treatment of fractures of the distal radius. Clin Orthop Relat Res 1986;(206): 202–10.

43. Jupiter JB. Fractures of the distal end of the radius. J Bone Joint Surg Am 1991;73(3):461–9.

44. Mekhail AO, Ebraheim NA, McCreath WA, et al. Anatomic and X-ray film studies of the distal articular surface of the radius. J Hand Surg Am 1996; 21(4):567–73.

45. Orbay JL, Fernandez DL. Volar fixation for dorsally displaced fractures of the distal radius: a preliminary report. J Hand Surg Am 2002;27(2):205–15.

46. Tirrell TF, Franko OI, Bhola S, et al. Functional consequence of distal brachioradialis tendon release: a biomechanical study. J Hand Surg Am 2013;38(5):920–6.

47. Ma T, Zheng X, He XB, et al. The role of brachioradialis release during AO type C distal radius fracture fixation. Orthop Traumatol Surg Res 2017; 103(7):1099–103.

48. Mann FA, Raissdana SS, Wilson AJ, et al. The influence of age and gender on radial height. J Hand Surg Am 1993;18(4):711–3.

49. Mignemi ME, Byram IR, Wolfe CC, et al. Radiographic outcomes of volar locked plating for distal radius fractures. J Hand Surg Am 2013;38(1):40–8.

50. Kamal RN, Shapiro LM. Practical application of the 2020 Distal Radius Fracture AAOS/ASSH Clinical Practice Guideline: a clinical Case. J Am Acad Orthop Surg 2022;30(9):e714–20.

51. Fernandez DL. Radial osteotomy and Bowers arthroplasty for malunited fractures of the distal end of the radius. J Bone Joint Surg Am 1988; 70(10):1538–51.

52. Hagert CG. Distal radius fracture and the distal radioulnar joint–anatomical considerations. Handchir Mikrochir Plast Chir 1994;26(1):22–6.

53. Slutsky DJ. External fixation of distal radius fractures. J Hand Surg Am 2007;32(10):1624–37.

54. Margaliot Z, Haase SC, Kotsis SV, et al. A meta-analysis of outcomes of external fixation versus plate osteosynthesis for unstable distal radius fractures. J Hand Surg Am 2005;30(6):1185–99.

55. Medoff RJ. Essential radiographic evaluation for distal radius fractures. Hand Clin 2005;21(3):279–88.

56. Kodama N, Takemura Y, Ueba H, et al. Acceptable parameters for alignment of distal radius fracture with conservative treatment in elderly patients. J Orthop Sci 2014;19(2):292–7.

57. Karnezis IA. Correlation between wrist loads and the distal radius volar tilt angle. Clin Biomech 2005;20(3):270–6.

58. Smith DW, Henry MH. Volar fixed-angle plating of the distal radius. J Am Acad Orthop Surg 2005; 13(1):28–36.

59. Lippross S. A technical note on the reduction of distal radius fractures with angular stable plates. J Orthop 2019;16(2):113–7.

60. Kapandji A. [Intra-focal pinning of fractures of the distal end of the radius 10 years later]. Ann Chir Main 1987;6(1):57–63.

61. Gui XY, Shi HF, Xiong J, et al. A modified intrafocal pinning technique with three-dimensional planning to facilitate volar plating in dorsally comminuted AO/OTA C2 and C3 distal radius fractures. BMC Musculoskelet Disord 2021;22(1):379.

62. Nauth A, McKee MD, Einhorn TA, et al. Managing bone defects. J Orthop Trauma 2011;25(8):462–6.

63. Ladd AL, Pliam NB. The role of bone graft and alternatives in unstable distal radius fracture treatment. Orthop Clin North Am 2001;32(2):337–51, ix.

64. Seiler JG, Johnson J. Iliac crest autogenous bone grafting: donor site complications. J South Orthop Assoc 2000;9(2):91–7.

65. Myeroff C, Archdeacon M. Autogenous bone graft: donor sites and techniques. J Bone Joint Surg Am 2011;93(23):2227–36.

66. Orbay JL, Badia A, Indriago IR, et al. The extended flexor carpi radialis approach: a new perspective for the distal radius fracture. Tech Hand Up Extrem Surg 2001;5(4):204–11.

67. Jupiter JB, Fernandez DL, Toh CL, et al. Operative treatment of volar intra-articular fractures of the distal end of the radius. J Bone Joint Surg Am 1996;78(12):1817–28.

68. Chin KR, Jupiter JB. Wire-loop fixation of volar displaced osteochondral fractures of the distal radius. J Hand Surg Am 1999;24(3):525–33.

69. Ruch DS, Yang C, Smith BP. Results of palmar plating of the lunate facet combined with external fixation for the treatment of high-energy compression fractures of the distal radius. J Orthop Trauma 2004;18(1):28–33.

70. Waters MJ, Ruchelsman DE, Belsky MR, et al. Headless bone screw fixation for combined volar lunate facet distal radius fracture and capitate fracture: case report. J Hand Surg Am 2014;39(8):1489–93.

71. Moore AM, Dennison DG. Distal radius fractures and the volar lunate facet fragment: Kirschner wire fixation in addition to volar-locked plating. Hand (N Y) 2014;9(2):230–6.

72. Gavaskar AS, Parthasarathy S, Balamurugan J, et al. Volar hook plate stabilization of volar marginal fragments in intra-articular distal radius fractures. Injury 2021;52(1):85–9.

73. Tordjman D, Hinds RM, Ayalon O, et al. Volar-ulnar approach for fixation of the volar lunate facet fragment in distal radius fractures: a technical tip. J Hand Surg Am 2016;41(12):e491–500.

Intraoperative Challenges in Hand Surgery

Doyle R. Wallace, MD*, Austin Luke Shiver, MD, Jonathon Whitehead, MD,
Matthew Wood, MD, Mark C. Snoddy, MD

KEYWORDS

• WALANT • Intraoperative resident education • Resource utilization

---

KEY POINTS

- Wide-awake local anesthesia no tourniquet (WALANT) is a popular technique, but achieving hemostasis and anesthesia can be challenging for certain procedures.
- Connecting traumatized patients to outpatient care can be a barrier, and coordinating care for polytraumatized patients adds complexity for all surgical providers involved.
- The order of multidisciplinary surgical procedures is influenced by patient complexity and institutional protocols.
- Intraoperative education for trainees in hand surgery faces challenges, and finding the right balance between the attending surgeon's involvement and trainees' experience is important.
- Operating room resources are sometimes limited for hand surgeons.

INTRODUCTION

Sterling Bunnell initiated the modern era of hand surgery when he published his seminal work *"Surgery of the Hand"* in 1944. As time has progressed, the practice of hand surgery has evolved and progressed as newer techniques have provided for a vast array of surgical interventions. As the innovations have changed the practice of hand surgery, various intraoperative challenges have presented themselves. This narrative seeks to identify some of the more common intraoperative challenges within the current scope of hand surgery. We intend to describe and elicit the uses and challenges of wide-awake surgery under local anesthesia without tourniquet, the barriers to operating on patients with hand/upper extremity trauma, elucidate particular operative challenges when surgeon learners are present, and finally, several resource limitations for hand surgeons.

DISCUSSION

Challenges in the Use of Wide-Awake Local Anesthesia No Tourniquet Surgery

The use of epinephrine with local analgesia for hemostasis is well described; however, since Bunnell's description in 1944 of epinephrine in the hand as a contraindication, the prevailing wisdom was to refrain from its use. With the critical reviews and experience of doctors Lalonde and Denkler, the advent of wide-awake local anesthesia no tourniquet surgery (WALANT) has become an accepted and viable alternative for practicing hand surgeons.[1,2] Benefits of WALANT have continued to be elucidated over the last 20 years with several representative categories including the ability to intervene on medically complex patients who would otherwise not tolerate a general anesthetic, decreased total clinical encounters, the ability to perform procedures at the time of initial consultation, avoidance of a fasting requirement, a decrease in required sterile supplies, decrease in medical resource utilization (anesthesia costs, preoperative and postoperative holding staffing) and overall cost, and the ability to test repair/fixation at the time of surgery.[3,4] WALANT is typically administered in a tumescent fashion with classic solution consisting of 1% lidocaine, 1:100,000 epinephrine mixed with a 1:20 ratio of 8.4% sodium bicarbonate. Lidocaine is typically dosed at a maximum dose of 7 mg/kg total dose. Our institution has had

---

Medical College of Georgia at Augusta University, 1120 15th Street, Augusta, GA 30912, USA
* Corresponding author.
E-mail address: dowallace@augusta.edu

Orthop Clin N Am 55 (2024) 123–128
https://doi.org/10.1016/j.ocl.2023.08.003

difficulty obtaining 1% lidocaine in recent months and as such substitutions have been made with 2% lidocaine when available as well as bupivacaine at a maximum dose of 3 mg/kg.

Although WALANT indications continue to expand and the practice has grown over the last quarter century, there still remain challenges to the use of this approach. Several issues arise when considering implementation in practice aiming to offer this method. First, one must consider the required timing for WALANT as compared to a more traditional local anesthesia with tourniquet or general anesthesia/monitored anesthesia care model. For maximum efficiency, local anesthesia with epinephrine requires approximately 30 minutes after injection for a hemostatic operative field.[5] As such, when planning for WALANT interventions, we recommend a similar approach to Dr Lalonde who recommends a dedicated block of time with multiple scheduled interventions, injecting the first 3 to 4 patients at the beginning of the allotted time followed by a rolling injection schedule.[3] Allowing for an appropriate time interval after injection will decrease the likelihood of conversion to a tourniquet or alternative anesthetic for a clear surgical field.

Second, provision should be made for the rare complication. Namely, supplies for basic life support should be readily available and serviceable, and staff should be regularly trained in their use. The antidote phentolamine should be kept on hand for digital ischemia, and lipid emulsion should be available for the rare and inadvertent injection of a large intravascular lidocaine load.[6]

Grandizio and colleagues surveyed 3826 members of the American Society for Surgery of the Hand with a 23% response rate and found that 62% of respondents utilized WALANT in some form or fashion in their current practice. Of note, 51% of respondents noted that an anesthesia provider was required at their institution. Specifically, when discussing reticence to the use of WALANT, 16% were concerned about appropriate visualization and 14% reported a simple unfamiliarity with the technique.[7] Unfamiliarity will certainly become less of a limiting factor as the practice expands and exposure during surgical training and fellowship becomes more commonplace. For the more mature surgeon, many resources exist as a reference for self-taught practice.[3,8]

Additional challenges to the use of WALANT entail visualization, patient cooperation, and patient anxiety. The primary prevention for appropriate visualization is timing after injection. As previously discussed, the optimal timing for a clear operative field is approximately 25 to 30 minutes after injection. For cases distal to the palmar digital crease, consideration can be given to a finger tourniquet if necessary, as an adjunct. With continued visualization needs proximal to the palmar digital crease, consideration should be given to aborting to a monitored anesthesia state or general anesthetic in the ambulatory surgery or hospital setting versus truncating the case if the patient is in the clinic setting with plans for a secondary procedure.

Patient cooperation and pre/intraprocedural anxiety remain issues best addressed prior to the procedure via patient selection. This selection ultimately relies on surgeon-based gestalt. When a patient is amenable to the WALANT technique but remains anxious, consideration can be given to provision of an appropriately dosed sedative (benzodiazepine) similar to patients requiring anxiolysis prior to advanced imaging. Additionally, patient anxiety regarding the injection and the required volume certainly remain a challenge to incorporation of WALANT. This can be ameliorated with the use of a small bore needle for the initial puncture, a perpendicular initial injection, and localizing the injection into palmar creases rather than glabrous skin. Finally, patient cooperation will continue to be a concern for the practitioner who practices WALANT. Clinical clues for cooperation entail close attention to clues from the social history (prompt follow-up, adherence to preoperative instructions, and prior interactions).

Connecting the Patient to the Hand Surgeon

Recognizing that the path to the operating room begins with entry into the health care system, hand and upper extremity trauma or pathology enters via a variety of entry points: emergency departments, outpatient nonspecialist clinics, urgent care clinics, and surgery clinics. Some of these environments may be highly skilled with a plethora of resources and clinician experience to accurately assess and properly triage these presenting pathologies. In contrast, other settings may lack the capability to provide the initial workup, diagnosis, and/or treatment and may require transfer to a higher level of care or referral for further follow-up.[9] In addition, specialist referral often requires recognition of surgical need by a nonsurgeon of wide specialty and experience.[10] Certainly, these nonsurgeon physicians and other providers are influenced by the facility they work in. Many health care facilities are not covered by a hand surgeon on call or are sometimes not easily referred within a health care system.[11]

Much of the transfer of care in an outpatient setting relies on the initial clinician's ability to communicate a surgical problem and the relative urgency of need. Furthermore, the transfer of records, images, and clinical findings within a single health care system is often complex. Patients themselves are often relied upon to shuttle clinical data that they themselves may not understand or appreciate. Systemic pathways must exist for capture of these surgical patients to provide adequate and timely care. Discharging surgical patients for outpatient follow-up removes the need for significant hospital and patient costs, but may not guarantee appropriate and timely connection to a hand specialist. Additionally, some institutions have multiple departments or groups that cover hand call-plastic surgery versus orthopedics versus general surgery, underscoring the reliance on clinicians who provide the initial triage for initial examination, temporization, and appropriate referral.

In our own level 1 trauma center, orthopedic trauma is primarily an inpatient service capturing a great deal of upper extremity and hand trauma in addition to acute infection and other pathology requiring inpatient admission. The affiliated hand team is available for assistance but often has a full outpatient surgery and clinic schedule, limiting nonemergent availability. In the polytraumatized patient, hand surgical coordination takes on an additional layer of complexity as multiple medical and surgical teams collaborate to provide care. As mentioned previously, upper extremity trauma is often reasonably immobilized while intra-abdominal, long bone fractures, and other more urgent surgical or medical issues are addressed. Thus, even at a level 1 trauma center, patients with surgical hand trauma or pathology require consistent coordination to provide proper care.

Ultimately, patients with surgical hand pathology must be connected to a capable hand surgeon for timely examination, accurate diagnosis, and appropriate surgical care. Significant barriers to this are inherent to patient care coordination and a complex health care system in addition to the wide variety of medical providers who initially triage these patients.

Challenges in Intraoperative Resident/Fellow Education

Surgical education is a challenge as it is a balance between the obligation of favorable patient care while balancing teaching and hands-on experience for the surgical trainee. One specific intraoperative challenge with resident education is the mix of residents in different stages of their career. All enter the hand operating room with different anatomic and procedural understanding as well as differences in surgical skill sets. Faculty must execute the steps of the case while trainees grasp the details of the case that are important to their level and understanding. While residents may have translatable skills from other services, they may be less developed with their exposure to soft tissue procedures, leaving them challenged by the innate nature of hand cases. Additionally, residents are only on the service for a limited time. Hand rotations are often spaced out in the time frame of years. Despite an advancement to upper-level resident status, there remains a learning curve to relearn the intraoperative specifics of a fine-tuned hand service. This makes it difficult for all residents to gain equal and fair exposure to more complicated cases if they are done infrequently. A combination of rare exposure to certain complex cases in conjunction with limited hands-on experience leads to the perpetuation of the need for advanced training in the form of fellowship.

During challenging cases, it can be difficult for a resident or fellow to execute crucial portions. The attending surgeon must ensure the case is performed safely and may hesitate to allow a trainee to complete key portions of the case, perhaps from lack of familiarity with the trainee's level of preparation or surgical skill. The art of the teaching surgeon is the ability to verbally communicate the goals and execution of the case without sacrificing the delivery of care from the training surgeon.

Additionally, the field of training also influences resident exposure and intraoperative skills within the field of hand surgery. Testa and colleagues analyzed such differences between the fields of plastic surgery and orthopedic surgery residency training. Their findings revealed plastics residents gained more exposure to nerve repairs and amputations as well as overall higher hand numbers. Orthopedics had a stronger exposure to bony trauma of the hand, wrist, and forearm.[12] These findings show that factors within interdepartmental training can influence intraoperative skills of trainees.

When considering ways to improve resident education, 1 aspect found especially useful in our department is the pre-case preparation review made by the resident before the case. This shows the resident is engaged and has given forethought to the steps of the procedure. In return, it helps establish an understanding of the indication for the surgery, key steps in the case, and vital structures encountered during the dissection, thus allowing for surgical educations catered to the trainee's level of understanding.

Setting expectations of trainees is vitally important to aid in intraoperative resident education. Before each case, there should be technical goals for the resident to perform. These should be level of training specific and tangible in provide realistic feedback. The attending surgeon should aim to find the time to share their thoughts in a post-case brief. During this time, it is helpful to talk about things that went well or maybe sources of difficulty. Attending physicians can bolster such discussions with guided reading before and after the case.

Challenges to Intraoperative Teams

Availability of intraoperative resources poses a challenge both in the hospital and ambulatory surgery center settings. A major challenge faced in the hospital setting is operating room inefficiencies. Efficiency in the operating room has become an area of focus for many hospitals due to its financial implications. Increasing procedural costs and reduced reimbursement rates have placed surgeons under increased pressure to improve productivity. A surgeon's efficiency is often limited by the constraints of perioperative and intraoperative factors, often outside the surgeon's control. Areas that are often inefficient are patient check-in, patient preparation, operating room turnover, anesthesia (including pre-procedure regional block), and surgical skills/surgeon behaviors.[13] Dedicated surgical teams have been identified as a way to mitigate intraoperative inefficiencies by reducing procedure time and turnover rate, improving communication, and maximizing overall patient safety.[14,15] Daniel and colleagues analyzed the turnover time between orthopedic and non-orthopedic-trained surgical technicians and circulating nurses. They found an overall significant reduction in turnover time between the 2 groups (30 minutes vs 20 minutes).[16]

Surgical familiarity has proven effective in total knee replacements as shown by Maruthappu and colleagues An evaluation of 4276 total knee replacements completed by 1163 different surgical teams revealed there was a direct correlation between operative time and team familiarity.[17] In addition to an improved efficiency, teams promote a sense of togetherness, identity, and team spirit lending to a more enjoyable work environment and ultimately improved patient care.[16]

There is a national trend toward travel nursing/surgical technicians leading to difficulties in assigning a cohesive surgical team for hand surgeons. Spontaneous assignment of surgical teams, nonpermanent staff ("travelers"), and intraoperative team turnover (lunch breaks, shift changes, and so forth.) have also been shown to increase operative times, interfere with communication, and disrupt the flow of surgery.[15] The limiting resource of a consistent intraoperative team poses a great challenge for hand surgery.

Intraoperative Imaging

Orthopedic hand surgeons are faced with the challenges of obtaining appropriate intraoperative imaging daily in both the outpatient and hospital settings. Obtaining intraoperative imaging requires successful patient positioning, appropriate imaging modalities, and often a skilled radiology technician. The list of necessary equipment required for patient positioning and intraoperative fluoroscopy is large: radiolucent operating beds or extremity positioners, arm boards/tables, bean bags or peg boards, fluoroscopy machines, and so forth. In the setting of increasing procedural costs and reduced reimbursement rates, the availability of the preferred/appropriate equipment and a skilled radiology technician is often limited. In addition, hand surgeons are often relegated to small operating rooms and are tasked with navigating large fluoroscopy machine in a small space. Sometimes these challenges can be mitigated by a mini-C arm, but its availability is not universal. Obtaining appropriate intraoperative imaging is vital in case execution and remains a great intraoperative challenge.

Issues with Hardware and Instrumentation in the Ambulatory Surgery Setting

Coordinating orthopedic implants plays a large role in the preoperative planning and intraoperative success. There are many implant options, each with their unique differences and clinical uses. Intraoperatively, a surgeon is often limited by the availability of certain implants or biologics. This limitation can be often magnified in the surgical center setting where the resources are limited due to the financial implications each product imposes on the facility. This limits a physician's ability to make "game time" decisions that veer from the preoperative plan and often increases operative time, reduces surgical success, and affects the overall patient outcome. This challenge may be moderated via thoughtful preoperative planning and coordination with ambulatory surgery centers.

Intraoperative Complication in the Ambulatory Setting

Intraoperative complications in the ambulatory surgery setting requiring an escalation of care can be devastating due to the lack of resources/ accommodations available to handle a higher level of acuity. An intraoperative consultation and available critical care unit are extremely valuable resources, specifically in upper extremity surgery when abnormal anatomy is frequently encountered. This poses a huge intraoperative challenge in the ambulatory surgery setting.

Goyal and colleagues looked at the safety of hand and upper extremity surgical procedures at a freestanding ambulatory surgery center. Of the 28,737 cases, there were a total of 58 adverse events (0.20%). Four patients were taken back to the operating room for bleeding complications, and 17 patients were transferred to the hospital immediately postoperatively: 6 for cardiac abnormalities, 3 for respiratory issues, 2 for uncontrolled hypertension, and the others for various other intraoperative concerns.[18] Though rare, the proximity of a hospital must be considered when performing surgery at an ambulatory surgery center.

A recent review suggests appropriate patient selection is vital in preventing complications, but the data guiding patient selection parameters and risk factors are limited and conflicting.[19] Though complications are rare, freestanding facilities with no ability to escalate care pose a huge intraoperative challenge to patient care.

CLINICS CARE POINTS

- Barriers to appropriate use of WALANT include inadequate time allotment to allow for hemostasis and poor patient selection given the need for patient cooperation as well as avoidance of anxiety.

- Upper extremity pathology can present to a variety of inpatient and outpatient clinical settings and practitioners; challenges connecting these patients to capable surgeons for appropriate and timely care must be addressed by consistent systemic and professional coordination.

- Intraoperative resident/fellow education is often challenged by the balance between the attending surgeon navigating appropriate patient care and granting the trainee adequate hands-on exposure.

- Resources limit the hand surgeon with a lack of personnel for dedicated surgical hand teams, implant limitations at ambulatory surgery centers, and obtaining appropriate intraoperative imaging.

ACKNOWLEDGMENTS

None.

CONFLICTS OF INTEREST

The authors have no conflicts of interest to declare. All co-authors have seen and agree with the contents of the manuscript and there is no financial interest to report. We certify that the submission is original work and is not under review at any other publication.

FUNDING

This research did not receive any specific grant from funding agencies in the public, commercial, or not-for-profit sectors.

REFERENCES

1. Lalonde D, Bell M, Benoit P, et al. A multicenter prospective study of 3,110 consecutive cases of elective epinephrine use in the fingers and hand: the Dalhousie Project clinical phase. J Hand Surg Am 2005;30(5):1061–7.
2. Thomson CJ, Lalonde DH, Denkler KA, et al. A critical look at the evidence for and against elective epinephrine use in the finger. Plast Reconstr Surg 2007;119(1):260–6.
3. Lalonde DH. Conceptual origins, current practice, and views of wide awake hand surgery. J Hand Surg 2017;42(9):886–95.
4. Connors KM, Guerra SM, Koehler SM. Current Evidence Involving WALANT Surgery. J Hand Surg Glob Online 2022;4(6):452–5.
5. McKee DE, Lalonde DH, Thoma A, et al. Achieving the optimal epinephrine effect in wide awake hand surgery using local anesthesia without a tourniquet. HAND 2015;10(4):613–5.
6. Rigney B, Casey C, McDonald C, et al. Distal radius fracture fixation using WALANT versus general and regional anesthesia: A systematic review and meta-analysis. Surgeon 2023;21(1):e13–22.
7. Grandizio LC, Graham J, Klena JC. Current trends in WALANT surgery: a survey of American Society for Surgery of the Hand members. Journal of Hand Surgery Global Online 2020;2(4):186–90.
8. Tan E, Bamberger HB, Saucedo J. Incorporating office-based surgery into your practice with WALANT. J Hand Surg 2020;45(10):977–81.
9. Patterson JM, Boyer MI, Ricci WM, et al. Hand trauma: a prospective evaluation of patients transferred to a level I trauma center. Am J Orthop 2010;39(4):196–200.
10. Hunt TJ, Powlan FJ, Renfro KN, et al. Common Finger Injuries: Treatment Guidelines for Emergency and Primary Care Providers. Mil Med 2023;022. https://pubmed.ncbi.nlm.nih.gov/36734106/.

11. Maroukis BL, Chung KC, MacEachern M, et al. Hand trauma care in the United States: a literature review. Plast Reconstr Surg 2016;137(1):100e.

12. Testa EJ, Orman S, Bergen MA, et al. Variability in Hand Surgery Training Among Plastic and Orthopaedic Surgery Residents. JAAOS Global Research & Reviews 2022;6(1).

13. Attarian DE, Wahl JE, Wellman SS, et al. Developing a high-efficiency operating room for total joint arthroplasty in an academic setting. Clin Orthop Relat Res 2013;471:1832–6.

14. Stepaniak PS, Vrijland WW, de Quelerij M, et al. Working with a fixed operating room team on consecutive similar cases and the effect on case duration and turnover time. Arch Surg 2010; 145(12):1165–70.

15. Kumar H, Morad R, Sonsati M. Surgical team: improving teamwork, a review. Postgrad Med 2019;95(1124):334–9.

16. Avery DM III, Matullo KS. The efficiency of a dedicated staff on operating room turnover time in hand surgery. J Hand Surg 2014;39(1):108–10.

17. Maruthappu M, Duclos A, Zhou CD, et al. The impact of team familiarity and surgical experience on operative efficiency: a retrospective analysis. J R Soc Med 2016;109(4):147–53.

18. Goyal KS, Jain S, Buterbaugh GA, et al. The safety of hand and upper-extremity surgical procedures at a freestanding ambulatory surgery center: a review of 28,737 cases. JBJS 2016;98(8):700–4.

19. Goldfarb CA, Bansal A, Brophy RH. Ambulatory surgical centers: a review of complications and adverse events. J Am Acad Orthop Surg 2017;25(1):12–22.

Foot and Ankle

Managing Intraoperative Fractures During Total Ankle Replacement

Christopher E. Gross, MD*, Daniel J. Scott, MD, MBA

KEYWORDS

- Total ankle complications • Periprosthetic fractures • Total ankle replacement

---

KEY POINTS

Intra-operative fractures are common and constant vigilance is needed to avoid fracture occurrence. A few specific technical tips are noted later in discussion.

- Avoiding over resection of the medial malleolus when choosing medial-lateral resection of the tibia
- Use of saw capture guides for the tibial and talar cuts, with special attention to medial-lateral resection when cutting the talus.
- Using caution and slow impaction if using a corner chisel on the tibial cut
- If a trial or definitive implant seems too wide medially or laterally, either downsize to a smaller implant, or use a reciprocating saw to gently widen the medial-lateral resection
- Impact the tibial component squarely in the coronal plane, without leaning medially or laterally

---

INTRODUCTION

Intraoperative complications during total ankle replacement (TAR) can be devastating.[1–4] As surgeons' experience with total ankles grow and surgical techniques are refined, intraoperative complications, such as fractures, can still occur. Surgeons must be able to recognize a problem, identify the options to remediate, and then execute a solution readily. Unfortunately, given the heterogeneity of TAR outcome studies, it is difficult to garner the true incidence of complications in the peri-operative period following ankle replacements. The purpose of this review is to focus on perioperative fractures during TAR. Fractures can occur intraoperatively and postoperatively as stress fractures or postoperative trauma. Periprosthetic fractures have been reported for every type of ankle implant design.[5]

In this article we seek to discuss complications and total ankle replacement as a whole, describe the types of intraoperative and postoperative fractures with total ankle, and provide an algorithm for the management of perioperative periprosthetic fractures.

Etiology of Intraoperative Fractures

Most intra-operative fractures are iatrogenic. They are often associated with inadequate exposure by the jig itself or size of the resection guide. Inadvertent use of the saw blade can cause fibula or medial malleolar fractures.

Medial malleolar fractures occur frequently due to the small bone bridge between the medial cortex and implant and can occur during the following surgical steps.

- Not checking medial-lateral positioning of cut guide after adjusting for sagittal or coronal balance
- Inadvertent saw blade cut while cutting talus through the jig
- Using a corner chisel to finish tibial cuts

Department of Orthopaedic Surgery, Medical University of South Carolina, 96 Jonathon Lucas Street, Charleston, SC 29425, USA
* Corresponding author.
E-mail address: cgross144@gmail.com

Orthop Clin N Am 55 (2024) 129–137
https://doi.org/10.1016/j.ocl.2023.05.013
0030-5898/24/© 2023 Elsevier Inc. All rights reserved.

- Removing corner chisel by levering off the medial malleolus
- Trialing implants that may be too tight to fit
- Impaction of tibial implant eccentrically

Lateral malleolar fractures occur much less commonly than medial malleolar fractures, with an intra-operative lateral malleolar fracture rate of roughly 14% of the rate of medial malleolar fractures.[6] However, they still occur at very specific times during an ankle replacement. Some 4th generation total ankle implants have a tibial component design that allows for the incinsura ([Exactech's Vantage [Gainesville, FL]; Cadence [Smith + Nephew, Watford, England]; Kinos [restor3d, Durham, NC]]) to facilitate a broader, tricortical footprint for the tibial component to be placed. During tibial bone preparation, the fibula is at tremendous risk when a surgeon needs to remove the entire lateral aspect of the tibia given then the fibula is recessed in its notch. The posterolateral border of the tibia cannot be sawed from the anterior aspect, but from the anteromedial aspect of the jig. (FIGURE)

Anterior or posterior tibial fractures can occur in patients during the impaction of the tibial baseplate.

Intra-operative talus fractures are an exceedingly rare complication of total ankle arthroplasty and can be of the neck or body. Talar neck fractures can occur in certain ankle systems in which the talar neck is removed for an anterior flange of a talar component. Another instance of increasing the risk of injuring the talus is in short necked talus and a chamfer is used when a flat top talus should have been, there by over-resecting the talar neck, increasing the talus fracture risk. The talar body is at risk for fracture during implantation.

Post-traumatic periprosthetic fractures of the ankle can result from forces that would have caused an injury to the region regardless of the presence of an implant, but also due to the inherent nature of the implantation process in general. Every total ankle system relies on pinning cutting guides and jigs into the tibia and talus. Therein, these small bicortical holes represent a significant iatrogenic stress riser that could weaken bone in mechanical loading. These holes raise the local stress in the region of the defect while the rest of the bone is relatively unperturbed by normal forces acting upon it. Up to 90% of periprosthetic fractures occur through a previously-made drill hole.[7] In a cadaveric study of 3.5 mm drill holes on the fibula,[8] the drilled fibulas failed at 59.6% of the mean load that was needed to fracture intact fibulas. A hole sized less then than 20% of the diameter of the bone can weaken the bone by 40% in bending and 12% in torsion.[9]

Post-operative pain following a TAR is a common etiology of patient dissatisfaction. Patients recovering from their arthroplasty have worsening pain and swelling at the 90 day timepoint postoperatively but then show gradual improvements in their function, pain, and range of motion for a year.[10] Patients who complain of persistent medial pain at the ankle have to be worked up and possibly treated for a stress fracture. At our institution, we check and correct any metabolic deficiencies, followed by imaging with a CT scan (FIGURE). We have tried Metal Artifact Reduction Sequences (MARS)-protocoled MRIs, but it did not give us the sensitivity needed to guide treatment. We have found some help in obtaining bone SPECT/CT scans to identify other potential sources of pain.[11]

In a study of 74 TAR performed by a single surgeon,[12] six patients who had persistent medial ankle pain at a mean of 12 months following index TAR underwent percutaneous placement of two medial malleolus screws drilled from the malleolar tip to proximal to the implant. VAS scores significantly improved in all patients. Interestingly, the average minimum width of the medial malleolus at the level of the tibial component was 2 mm thinner in those who had medial pain than a control group (10.2 vs 12.2 mm, $P < .05$) and there were no radiographic signs of medial malleolar stress injury. Doets and colleagues reported on mobile-bearing devices in 93 patients with inflammatory arthritis.[13] Four patients developed atraumatic fractures of the distal tibia at the level of the tip of the stem of the tibia component. It was noted intra-operatively that these patients had severe osteopenia. All were treated successfully with cast immobilization.

A prospective collected database of 194 ankles was screened for all periprosthetic fractures.[14] Seven intraoperative and 9 postoperative periprosthetic fractures were identified (3.5% and 4.5%, respectively). Seven patients (3.5% of total or 43.8% of all fractures) underwent TAR removal or revision. Lower tibial and talar Hounsfield units (HU, a measure of bone radio density derived from a computer tomography scan), lower weight, and lower BMI were associated with periprosthetic fractures. Once the researchers controlled for age, sex, and weight, only a decreased tibial HU was significantly associated with periprosthetic fracture.

All intraoperative fractures occurred in patients with tibial HU less than 200.

Incidence

In an evidence-based classification of complications in total ankle replacement,[15] intraoperative fractures and wound healing problems are considered low-grade complications in TAR. Technical error, subsidence of the implant and postoperative periprosthetic fracture are considered medium grade complications. The high-grade complications included deep infection, aseptic loosening, and implant failure. The level of danger a particular complication achieved was based on if it caused surgical failure greater than 50%, less than 50%, or rarely. The 20 studies that met inclusion criteria, intraoperative fractures caused 0% of implant failure and an incidence of 8.1%. This was the third most common complication surrounding an ankle replacement surgery. Fractures after a total ankle replacement occurred in 5% of individuals which led to 16.7% of the rate of failure the given complication.

There are two recent systematic literature reviews and meta-analyses regarding complications following total ankle arthroplasty.[16,17] In a systematic review which reported on 16,000, 964 ankles average follow-up of 48 months,[16] the highest complication was an intraoperative fracture (5.6%), followed by impingement. In their meta-analysis, they demonstrated a fracture rate of 4.9% of the medial malleolus and 1.7% of the lateral malleolus. Of all the fractures listed, 77% of them were fixed during the index surgery. Postoperative fractures occurred roughly 4.0% of the time. In another systematic review of 4412 ankles,[17] intraoperative fractures occurred roughly 2.8% of the time, while postoperative fractures occurred in 1.3% of all total ankle replacements.

In a study of a 505 TARs from a single center over 10 years of a single implant, a total of 21 patients with a periprosthetic fracture were identified.[5] There were 11 intra-operative and ten post-operative fractures. Of the eight stress fractures, five were treated conservatively and the remaining three were treated operatively. Patients who had intraoperative ankle fractures had statistically better patient-reported outcome (PROs) measures than those who had stress or post-traumatic fractures, though their pain scores were the same. All patients achieved union, though 3 (14.3%) had delayed union.

A Treatment Algorithm

We recommend the immediate and primary fixation of intra-operative periprosthetic fractures.

This allows normal post-operative osseous integration of the prosthesis and routine early rehabilitation. We believe that this decreases implant loosening or subsidence. Furthermore, the risk of nonunion is minimized.

Avoiding Intra-operative Fractures

Intra-operative fractures are common and constant vigilance is needed to avoid fracture occurrence. A few specific technical tips are noted later in discussion.

- Fluoroscopic verification of medial-lateral positioning of tibial cut guide after adjusting for sagittal or coronal balance
- Avoiding over resection of the medial malleolus when choosing medial-lateral resection of the tibia
- Use of saw capture guides for the tibial and talar cuts, with special attention to medial-lateral resection when cutting the talus.
- Using caution and slow impaction if using a corner chisel on the tibial cut
- When removing the corner chisel, try to either pull the chisel straight out, or if anything lever inferiorly. A back-slap on the corner chisel can be useful to help with this step.
- If a trial or definitive implant seems to wide medially or laterally, either downsize to a smaller implant, or use a reciprocating saw to gently widen the medial-lateral resection
- Impact the tibial component squarely in the coronal plane, without leaning medially or laterally

Treatment of Medial Malleolar Fractures

Medial malleolar fractures are the most commonly encountered intra-operative fracture.[3,5,18] Most commonly, these occur during oscillating saw use while resecting the distal tibia, or less commonly during tibial component impaction. All intra-operative medial malleolus fractures should be stabilized to allow for maximal prosthesis integration, appropriate ligamentous balancing, and to reduce the risk of any future medial malleolar stress injuries.

Of note, in an analysis of bone tension during the fixation of an intraoperative medial malleolus fracture,[19] a finite element study based on CT examinations demonstrated that fracture fixation using a Blount staple leads to lowest bone tension (by half) around the fixation of the medial malleolus versus a screw or staple and screw construct. However, good results have been reported with the use of cannulated screw fixation, as well as less commonly plate fixation. All approaches are reasonable and typically have high associated rates of union.

Figs. 1–3 are the intra-operative and post-operative radiographs of an intra-operative medial malleolus fracture treated with cannulated screw fixation. Fig. 4 shows a 6 week post-operative X-rays of an uncomplicated total ankle (see Fig. 4), which sustained a medial malleolar fracture at 3 months post-operative, seen on X-ray and CT (Figs. 5 and 6 respectively). This was treated with a medial distal tibial locking plate (Fig. 7) which went on to un-eventful union (Fig. 8 shows a post-operative CT scan)

Treatment of Lateral Malleolar Fractures

Peri-prosthetic fibular fractures are likely the second most common intra-operative peri-prosthetic fracture behind medial malleolar fractures.[3,5,18] Intra-operative fibular fractures are thought to most commonly occur while using an oscillating saw to create either the initial tibial or talar cut. Less commonly, fibular fractures can occur from during the insertion of the tibial component if the medial to lateral distance of the tibial component is wider than the resected bone. The vast majority of inter-operative fibular fractures are unstable and warrant stabilization, allowing for maximal prosthesis inter-osseous integration. Most commonly this is performed through open reduction and internal fixation via a direct lateral approach and fixated with a plate. The majority of these fractures tend to

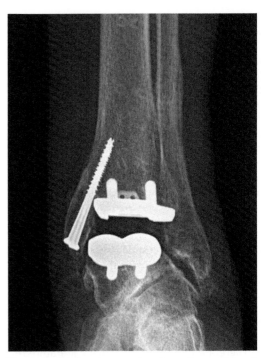

Fig. 2. Weightbearing mortise view of a medial malleolar fracture fixed with cannulated screws.

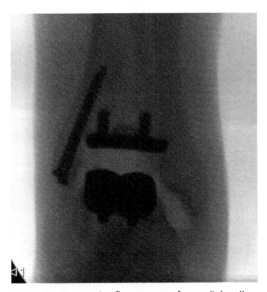

Fig. 1. Intra-operative fluoroscopy of a medial malleolar fracture fixed with cannulated screws.

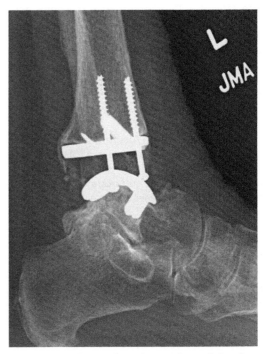

Fig. 3. Weightbearing lateral view of a medial malleolar fracture fixed with cannulated screws.

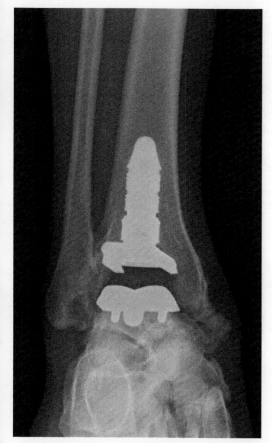

Fig. 4. Post-operative weightbearing ankle radiograph after total ankle replacement.

be transverse in nature, and a locking plate can sometimes be useful, as the fibula fractures can sometimes be fairly distal on the fibula. Occasionally, in more proximal fractures, a fibular nail can also be used as an alternative to a plate.

Figs. 9 and 10 show a typical case of an intra-operative distal fibular fracture treated with open reduction and internal fixation with a distal fibular locking plate. This went on to un-eventful union as shown in Figs. 11 and 12.

Treatment of Talus Fractures

Inter-operative talus fractures are less common than medial malleolus and fibular fractures and can be more challenging to manage.[5,16,18,20] Intra-operatively, these fractures most commonly occur during the impaction of the talar component. The surgeon should ensure that either the implant is stable prior to proceeding with fracture fixation, or if the implant has not yet been fully impacted, then the fracture should be fixated first then the implant fully seated. In some instances, revision of the talar

component may be necessary to ensure talar stability and correct talar position.

One of the more common patterns of talar fracture is a talar neck fracture, which is often transverse and occurs just distal to the anterior flange of the talar component during impaction. Talar fracture are almost always unstable and require stabilization. This is most commonly performed by extending the anterior approach to the tala-navicular joint and opening the talar navicular joint. This allows for the placement of anterior to posterior screws from the talar head into the talar body, stabilizing a talar neck fracture. A sinus tarsi incision can also be created if either better visualization of the reduction is needed or if the placement of a lateral plate, though this is usually not required.

Treatment of Post-op Fractures

Periprosthetic fractures can be challenging to treat for both the surgeon and patient. Lazarides

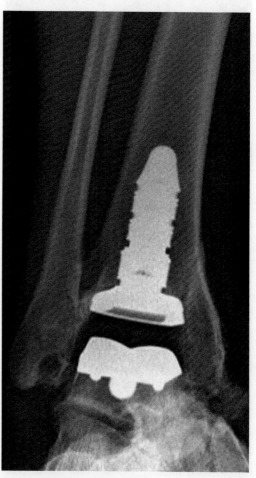

Fig. 5. Weightbearing mortise view of a post-operative medial malleolus fracture.

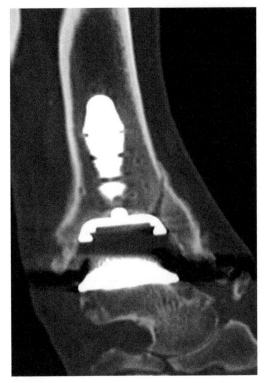

Fig. 6. Coronal computer tomography view of a post-operative medial malleolar fracture.

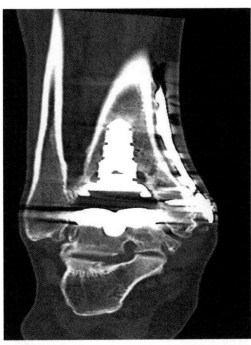

Fig. 8. Coronal computer tomography view of post-operative medial malleolar fracture treated with a medial locking plate which went on to union.

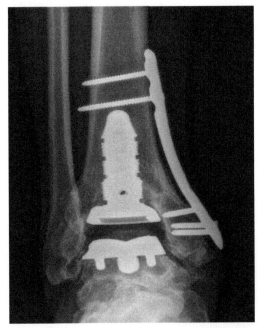

Fig. 7. Weightbearing mortise view of a post-operative medial malleolus fracture treated with a medial locking plate.

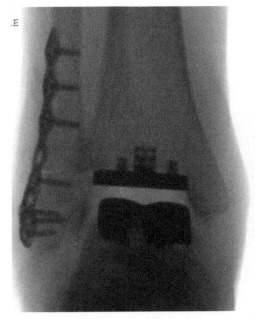

Fig. 9. Intra-operative fluoroscopic mortise view of a distal fibular fracture fixed with a locking plate.

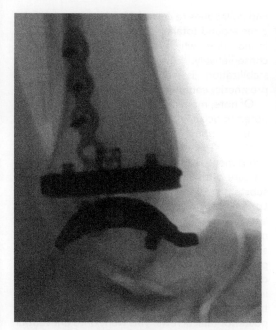

Fig. 10. Intra-operative fluoroscopic lateral view of a distal fibular fracture fixed with a locking plate.

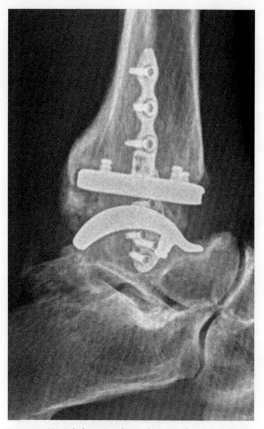

Fig. 12. Weightbearing lateral view of a distal fibular fracture fixed with a locking plate.

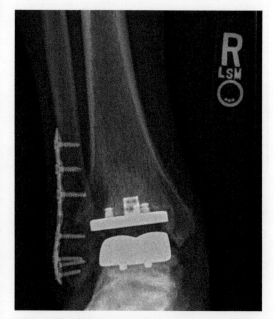

Fig. 11. Weightbearing mortise view of a distal fibular fracture fixed with a locking plate.

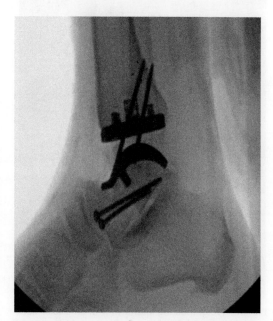

Fig. 13. Intra-operative fluoroscopic lateral view of a talar neck fracture treated with solid screw fixation.

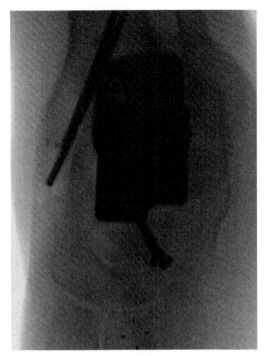

Fig. 14. Intra-operative anterior to posterior foot view of a talar neck fracture treated with solid screw fixation.

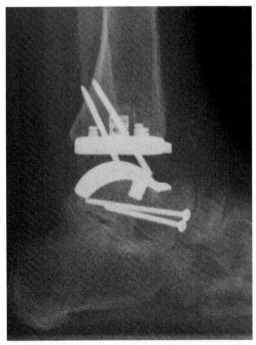

Fig. 15. Weightbearing lateral view of an a talar neck fracture treated with solid screw fixation which went on to union.

and colleagues reviewed 32 post-operative fractures around total ankle arthroplasties, and only found one which was successfully treated conservatively.[20] Given these findings, surgical stabilization is recommended for all peri-prosthetic, complete fractures.

Of note, medial malleolus fractures have been noted to occur in the early post-operative period in association with varus position of the tibial implant.[5] This is varus mal-position of the tibial component is thought to cause an insufficiency fracture of the medial malleolus.[5] When there is substantial varus mal-position of the tibial component in the coronal plane, this is likely best treated with either a corrective supra-malleolar osteotomy or tibial component revision. Other medial malleolar fractures in the early post-operative period are likely best treated with definitive stabilization. **Figs. 13** and **14** show an intra-operative talar neck fracture which was treated with stabilization with two anterior to posterior talar screws. This went onto uneventful union as shown in **Fig. 15**.

CLINICS CARE POINTS

- Most intra-operative fractures are iatrogenic. They are often associated with inadequate exposure by the jig itself or size of the resection guide.
- Inadvertent use of the saw blade can cause fibula or medial malleolar fractures.
- When planning the width of the implant, please consider the width of the medial malleolus as one does not want to leave less than 11mm.
- Lateral malleolar fractures occur much less frequently than medial malleolar fractures; they still occur at very specific times during an ankle replacement.
- Patients who complain of persistent medial pain at the ankle have to be worked up and possibly treated for a stress fracture.

DISCLOSURE

The authors have nothing to disclose.

REFERENCES

1. Borenstein TR, Anand K, Li Q, et al. A Review of Perioperative Complications of Outpatient Total Ankle Arthroplasty. Foot Ankle Int 2018;39(2): 143–8.

2. Heida KA, Waterman B, Tatro E, et al. Short-Term Perioperative Complications and Mortality After Total Ankle Arthroplasty in the United States. Foot Ankle Spec 2018;11(2):123–32.

3. Myerson MS, Mroczek K. Perioperative complications of total ankle arthroplasty. Foot Ankle Int 2003;24(1):17–21.

4. Williams JR, Wegner NJ, Sangeorzan BJ, Brage ME. Intraoperative and perioperative complications during revision arthroplasty for salvage of a failed total ankle arthroplasty. Foot Ankle Int 2015;36(2):135–42.

5. Tsitsilonis S, Schaser KD, Wichlas F, et al. Functional and radiological outcome of periprosthetic fractures of the ankle. Bone Joint J 2015;97:950–6.

6. Clough TM, Alvi F, Majeed H. Total ankle arthroplasty: what are the risks?: a guide to surgical consent and a review of the literature. Bone Joint Lett J 2018;100-B(10):1352–8.

7. Koval KJ FV, Kummer F, Green S. Complications of fracture fixation devices. In: CH Epps J Jr, editor. Complications in orthopaedic surgery. Philadelphia: Lippincott; 1994. p. 131–54.

8. Johnson BA, Fallat LM. The effect of screw holes on bone strength. J Foot Ankle Surg 1997;36(6):446–51.

9. Laurence M, Freeman MA, Swanson SA. Engineering considerations in the internal fixation of fractures of the tibial shaft. J Bone Joint Surg Br 1969;51(4):754–68.

10. Pagenstert G, Horisberger M, Leumann AG, et al. Distinctive pain course during first year after total ankle arthroplasty: a prospective, observational study. Foot Ankle Int 2011;32(2):113–9.

11. Mertens J, Lootens T, Vercruysse J, et al. Bone SPECT/CT in the Evaluation of Painful Total Ankle Replacement: Validation of Localization Scheme and Preliminary Evaluation of Diagnostic Patterns. Clin Nucl Med 2021;46(5):361–8.

12. Lundeen GA, Dunaway LJ. Etiology and Treatment of Delayed-Onset Medial Malleolar Pain Following Total Ankle Arthroplasty. Foot Ankle Int 2016;37(8):822–8.

13. Doets HC, Brand R, Nelissen RG. Total ankle arthroplasty in inflammatory joint disease with use of two mobile-bearing designs. J Bone Joint Surg Am 2006;88(6):1272–84.

14. Cody EA, Lachman JR, Gausden EB, et al. Lower Bone Density on Preoperative Computed Tomography Predicts Periprosthetic Fracture Risk in Total Ankle Arthroplasty. Foot Ankle Int 2019;40(1):1–8.

15. Glazebrook MA, Arsenault K, Dunbar M. Evidence-based classification of complications in total ankle arthroplasty. Foot Ankle Int 2009;30(10):945–9.

16. Hermus JP, Voesenek JA, van Gansewinkel EHE, et al. Complications following total ankle arthroplasty: A systematic literature review and meta-analysis. Foot Ankle Surg 2022;28(8):1183–93.

17. Vale C, Almeida JF, Pereira B, et al. Complications after total ankle arthroplasty- A systematic review. Foot Ankle Surg 2023;29(1):32–8.

18. Manegold S., Haas N.P., Tsitsilonis S., et al., Periprosthetic fractures in total ankle replacement: classification system and treatment algorithm. J Bone Joint Surg Am. 2013;95(9):815-820, S1-3.

19. Lorkowski J, Wilk R, Pokorski M. In Silico Analysis of Bone Tension During Fixation of the Medial Malleolus Fracture After Ankle Joint Endoprosthesis. Adv Exp Med Biol 2021;1335:103–9.

20. Lazarides AL, Vovos TJ, Reddy GB, et al. Algorithm for Management of Periprosthetic Ankle Fractures. Foot Ankle Int 2019;40(6):615–21.

Spine

Intraoperative Vertebral Artery Injury
Evaluation, Management, and Prevention

Nathan Redlich, MD[a],*, Daniel Gelvez, MD[a],
Katherine Dong, MD[a], Matthew Darlow, MD[a],
Jestin Williams, MD[a], Berje Shammassian, MD[b],
Amit K. Bhandutia, MD[c]

KEYWORDS

- Cervical spine • Vertebral artery injury • Iatrogenic complications • Vertebral artery anomaly
- Intraoperative management • Surgical technique

KEY POINTS

- Iatrogenic vertebral artery injury (VAI) is a rare but potentially devastating complication of cervical spine surgery.
- Prevention is key to avoiding any injury through knowledge of patient anatomy, procedure and instrumentation selection, care in dissection, and meticulous surgical technique.
- Initial management of VAI includes tamponade and enlistment of anesthesia assistance in addition to neurointerventional radiology/surgery or vascular surgery if available.
- Surgeons must be aware of late complications of VAI and management options.

INTRODUCTION

Vertebral artery injury (VAI) is the most common vascular injury during cervical spine surgery and makes up 86.6% of iatrogenic cervical spine vascular injuries.[1] The typical mechanism of VAI in cervical spine surgery is laceration. The most common causes are drilling (anterior approach) and instrumentation (posterior approach). Delayed complications from arterial laceration include recurrent bleeding, pseudoaneurysm development, and arteriovenous fistula (AVF) formation.[2] Neurologic complications from VAI are rare (5%) but can result in potentially devastating ischemia or cerebral infarct due to thrombosis with subsequent emboli.[1] The risk of these complications depends on VA dominance, baseline health of the patient, and management of the injury. Once hemorrhage is controlled patients may frequently be asymptomatic from these injuries, but the possibility of late neurologic sequelae cannot be ignored. The authors would highlight the primary importance of prevention in knowledge of individual patient anatomy, careful selection of procedure choice, and instrumentation techniques to reduce the likelihood of VAI.

ANATOMY

Knowledge of VA anatomy and prevalence of anomalies is critical to avoid iatrogenic injury to this artery. The traditionally described anatomy of the VA is that of 4 arterial segments (Fig. 1). The extraosseous origin (V1) branches from the subclavian artery and travels anterior to the C7 transverse process to the entry point of the C6 transverse foramen (TF). The artery then passes within the TF of C6 to the TF of the axis (V2). Most traumatic injuries to the VA occur in segment V2 due to close proximity during

---

[a] LSUHSC Orthopaedic Surgery Resident, 2021 Perdido Street, 7th Floor, New Orleans, LA 70112, USA; [b] LSUHSC Neurosurgery, 2021 Perdido Street, 7th Floor, New Orleans, LA 70112, USA; [c] LSUHSC Orthopaedic and Spine Surgery, 2021 Perdido Street, 7th Floor, New Orleans, LA 70112, USA
* Corresponding author.
E-mail address: nredli@lsuhsc.edu

Orthop Clin N Am 55 (2024) 139–149
https://doi.org/10.1016/j.ocl.2023.06.006
0030-5898/24/Published by Elsevier Inc.

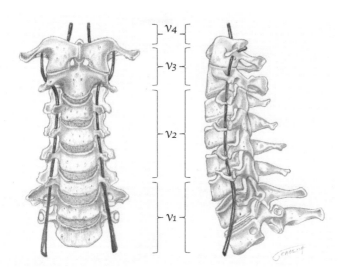

Fig. 1. Vertebral artery anatomy. Left: coronal view of the vertebral artery segments labeled V1–V4. Right: sagittal view of the course of the vertebral artery through the transverse foramina of the vertebrae.

drilling, tapping, and insertion of lateral mass or pedicle screws. After passing through the TF of the axis, the artery courses laterally and superiorly through the TF of the atlas then along the posterolateral aspect of the ring of C1(V3) until perforating the posterior atlantoaxial membrane to the foramen magnum. At this level, the VA is vulnerable during lateral exposure and laminectomy of C1. Intradural extension of the artery (V4) continues to unite with the contralateral VA forming the basilar artery that supplies the brain stem and cerebellum.

Anomalies must be identified before surgery to avoid inadvertent VAI. The incidence of anomalous VA ranges from 2.7% in cadaveric studies to 5.4% in imaging studies.[3,4] Assessment with computed tomography angiogram (CTA) or magnetic resonance angiogram (MRA) highlights anatomic features including vessel course and characterization. Anomalies typically fall within 3 categories: extraforaminal anomalies, intraforaminal anomalies, and arterial anomalies.

Extraforaminal anomalies occur when the artery is found anterior to the foramen rather than within its respective TF from C6-C2 (Fig. 2A). Several studies have found a 93% to 95% incidence of VA entry into TF at C6.[4,5] When entering the TF cephalad to C6, the artery runs unprotected just beneath the longus colli muscle posing a risk with muscle reflection during an anterior cervical approach.

Intraforaminal abnormalities involve midline migration and often a tortuous course of the artery (Fig. 2B). A cadaveric study of cervical spines defined an anomalous artery as the presence of the foramen transversariurm either medial or less than 1.5 mm lateral to the uncovertebral joint.[3] Some authors propose that an acute injury may lead to the development of a tortuous VA, whereas others describe a degenerative process in which the artery becomes tortuous causing erosion of the posterolateral aspects of the vertebral body.[6] Eskander and colleagues[6] found a significant association between older age and the presence of medially migrating arteries, hypothesizing that midline migration may be a chronic degenerative osteoarthritic process. Furthermore, several studies have shown the left VA to more often migrate medially than the right which may be a consequence of left sided dominance.[3,6] Medial migration of the artery may impact the surgeon's ability to safely perform lateral decompression and removal of uncovertebral joint when required.

Arterial anomalies include fenestrated, duplicated, or hypoplastic arteries (Fig. 2C). Congenital variants of VA anatomy can exist, most notably arterial dominance. Traditionally, VA dominance has been considered as a finding with little clinical significance; however, recent studies have shown hypoplasia to be a risk factor for posterior circulation stroke.[7] Some studies have found left dominance in 64% to 73% of the healthy population, whereas other studies have found minor differences.[4,8] Understanding these abnormalities can alert the surgeon to risk of VAI and potential for neurologic sequelae. Notable variants at the C1-2 level include persistent first intersegmental artery as the most common variant (3%), fenestration of the C1 (1%), and posterior inferior cerebellar artery originating at C1-2(1%). These variants can be

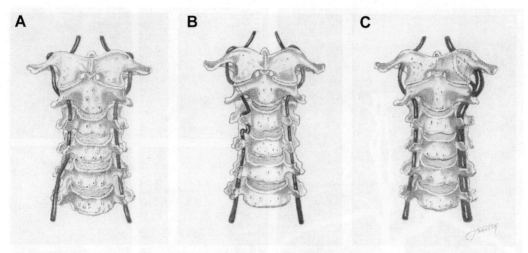

Fig. 2. Vertebral artery anomalies. (*A*) Extraforaminal anomaly depicted by VA entrance into the transverse foramen at C4. (*B*) Intraforaminal anomaly depicted by a tortuous course of the right VA with medialization of the artery at the C3 vertebral body. (*C*) Arterial anomalies depicted by a dominant left VA and an anomalous medialized fenestration at C1.

unilateral or bilateral.[9] Meticulous review of the preoperative angiogram for risk assessment of the VA is critical for a safe spine procedure (**Fig. 3**). If an anomaly is identified preoperatively, the surgeon may elect for cervical discectomy rather than corpectomy at the level of the anomaly or even consider a posterior approach to the cervical spine.

PREVENTION
Preoperative Imaging
Preoperative planning is essential to avoiding VAIs. Almost all patients undergoing a cervical spine procedure will have a preoperative MRI or CT scan that requires careful review. Both preoperative imaging modalities allow for measuring of appropriate screw length within the bony confines of the cervical spine. However, the course of the VA itself is just as important as the bony anatomy. Although angiography may not be necessary for typical anterior cervical procedures or lateral mass screws, surgeons should use vascular imaging modalities such as CT angiography or MR angiography in patients undergoing C1 or C2 instrumentation. Other indications for obtaining advanced imaging with angiography could include anatomic abnormalities discussed in the prior section. These variations may be noted on MRI or inferred from bony anatomy on CT scan. For example, an abnormally expanded TF may be indicative of a tortuous VA with medial loops or a high riding course and prompt further investigation with angiography. Another example would be a VA

that enters above the C6 TF leaving the more caudal part of the artery exposed to injury during an anterior approach. A hypoplastic TF at C6 or C5 should raise suspicion for this variant.[10]

At the atlantoaxial spine, angiography of the VA may influence the fixation technique employed by the surgeon: C1/2 transarticular screw, C2 pedicle screw, C2 pars screw, or C2 translaminar screws. The path of the VA will largely determine the use of fixation. If a high riding VA is found creating a narrow bony channel in the sagittal plane, transarticular C1/2 screw fixation may not be a viable option.[11] Notably, independent fixation of C1 lateral mass and C2 pedicle screws are generally safer than placement of C1/2 transarticular screws.[12] The authors prefer the use of the Goel-Harms technique using independent fixation of C1 and C2 rather than the C1/2 transarticular screw for this reason and reserve use of the transarticular screw for limited indications. A high riding VA or small pedicle will generally preclude the use of the stronger pedicle screw and use of the pars or translaminar screw may be more judicious. It must be noted that the pars screw trajectory aims directly at the path of the VA as it exits the C2 vertebra and thus can still result in injury. The path of the C2 pedicle screw starts at its most dangerous point near the VA; it is angled away from the path of the VA as it crosses the junction of the posterior aspect of C2 into the anterior body. In addition, the C2 screw has the prerequisite of an intact posterior arch and planning to place bilateral screws.

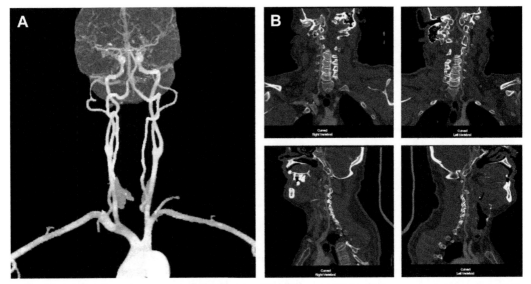

Fig. 3. Vertebral artery codominance on preoperative CT angiogram. (*A*) Codominant vertebral arteries. (*B*) Top images demonstrate coronal views of patent codominant vertebral arteries; bottom images demonstrate sagittal views of patent codominant vertebral arteries.

Classification Systems

A VA classification system proposed by Eskander and colleagues[6] is a useful tool to surgeons for the purpose of preoperative planning (Fig. 4). Three zones are described: zone 1 (lateral to the uncovertebral joint), zone 2 (at the level of the uncovertebral joint), and zone 3 (medial to the uncovertebral joint). It is a modification of the radiographic grading system developed by Oga and colleagues[13] to evaluate artery tortuosity described in 4 types: Type 1, the artery is straight in zone 1; Type 2, the artery is mildly tortuous in zone 1; Type 3, the artery has loop formation with the medial portion in zone 2; Type 4, the artery has loop formation in zone 3. Based on MRI, the Eskander and colleagues[6] grading system accounts for arterial abnormalities such as arterial hypoplasia or fenestration. Standardization of this grading system enables surgeons to detect and grade VA anomalies in an organized manner with respect to intraforaminal midline migration, extraforaminal altered TF entrance, and arterial dominance.

APPROACH AND INSTRUMENTATION
Anterior Cervical Spine

The VA is at risk during the anterior approach to the subaxial cervical spine due to its anatomic location in the C2 through C6 transverse foramina (Fig. 5). It lies just lateral to the uncovertebral joints that lie at the lateral margins of the operative field in anterior cervical spine procedures. Care must be taken during dissection to stay midline on the cervical spine that generally can be identified in between the longus colli. In patients with severe degenerative disease, care should be taken when removing osteophytes, particularly near C6-7 or near an extraforaminal VA. Exposure of the anterior cervical spine should include visualization of the uncovertebral joints. Use of a penfield dissector beneath the longus colli while retracting along the outside of the uncus can allow for dissection of the anterior cervical spine to visualize the uncus safely. Bipolar electrocautery is recommended over monopolar electrocautery due to the risk of inadvertent damage to the VA. Identification

Type	Tortuosity	Migration
1	Straight	Zone 1
2	Mildly tortuous	Zone 1
3	Loop formation	Zone 2
4	Loop formation	Zone 3

Modifier	Arterial Abnormality
A	Normal (equal or <2mm size differential)
B	Abnormal (hypoplastic/absent or fenestrated arteries)

Fig. 4. Classification of vertebral artery (VA) tortuosity as described by Oga and colleagues (*left*) and modified by Eskander and colleagues (*right*).

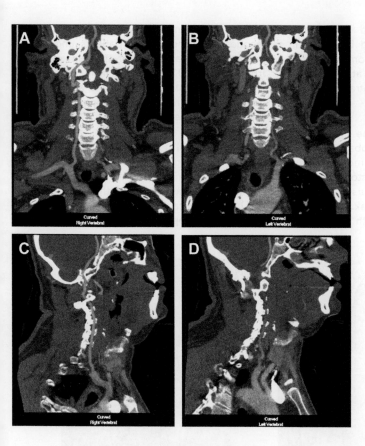

Fig. 5. Postoperative computed tomography angiogram (CTA) after intraoperative left vertebral artery injury showing occlusion of the left vertebral artery with retrograde flow. (*A*) Coronal view of patent intact right vertebral artery. (*B*) Coronal view of injured left vertebral artery. (*C*) Sagittal view of patent intact right vertebral artery. (*D*) Sagittal view of injured left vertebral artery.

of the uncus will allow the surgeon to stay within the "goal posts," particularly during corpectomy procedure. The technique is generally protective against oblique corpectomy troughs that can stray into the path of the VA, particularly at the middle third of the vertebral body. In addition, care should be taken to work away from the VA in working lateral to medial. In the event of uncinate resection, a penfield dissector can be placed lateral to the uncus to allow for protection of the VA. Despite its proximity to the operative field, injury to the VA during the anterior cervical exposure remains rare, occurring at a rate 0.18% to 0.5%.[14]

Atlantoaxial Spine

According to a systematic review of 11 studies by Ghaith and colleagues[15] evaluating posterior atlantoaxial instrumentation, the rate of VAI was 2% per patient among 773 patients and 1% per screw placed among 2238 screws placed. Knowledge of the VA and its path is paramount in exposure and instrumentation. As detailed in the section above, preoperative planning is ideal for selecting the type of instrumentation at the C1-2 level. Prior to placement of instrumentation, dissection is of paramount importance.

At the C1 level, dissecting more than 1.5 cm lateral from midline places the most cephalad aspect VA at risk.[3] In 15% of patients there is a bony bridge over this aspect of the VA rather than a true foramen called the ponticulus posticus which also should be considered during dissection to avoid injury.[16] This anatomic structure may be mistaken for the posterior arch and inadvertent dissection may result in direct injury to the artery. At the C1 and C2 levels judicious use of the cobb elevator, periosteal elevator, or penfield dissector will allow for a gentle blunt sweeping of tissues. When approaching the border of the safe zone, it is recommended to switch to use of bipolar electrocautery for better control of the field. As emphasized previously, careful use of screw selection will help to avoid injury to the VA. The authors will use fluoroscopy in placement of C2 screws to ensure trajectory matches that previously planned on CT imaging. In addition, multiplanar reconstruction on CT imaging can allow for care planning of C2 screws. In placement of C2 pedicle screws, exposure of the medial border of the pedicle will allow for angling of the screw medially while avoiding injury to the spinal cord due to direct visualization. This medial exposure can be performed with an angled curette or Penfield #1 dissector. In addition, consideration should be made in instrumenting the side with nondominant VA in case of vascular injury—this will at least allow for unilateral fixation if the contralateral side cannot be instrumented (Fig. 6).

Posterior Subaxial Cervical Spine

In the posterior approach to the subaxial cervical spine, lateral mass screws are the most common method of fixation. If the trajectory of these screws is too medial, the VA coursing through the transverse foramina is at risk. This is an exceedingly rare complication with lateral mass

screws. A systematic review by Coe and colleagues[17] looking at 758 patients undergoing posterior cervical fusion of the subaxial spine from 1980 to 2011 found no incidences of VAI. However, this structure remains an important consideration when instrumenting this area of the cervical spine.

INTRAOPERATIVE MANAGEMENT

Surgical Technique in Event of Injury

Initial hemostatic tamponade

In the event of vascular injury, the initial response will have significant downstream consequences. Control of the operating room is of the utmost

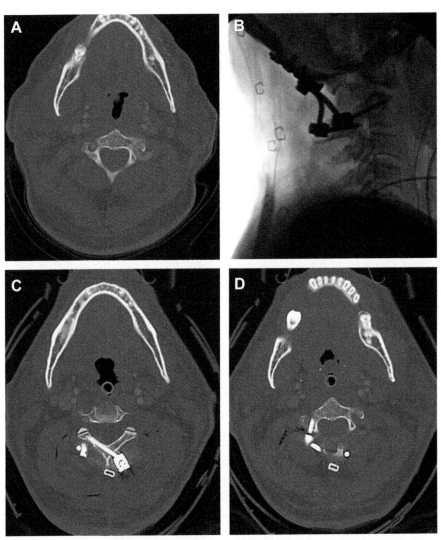

Fig. 6. Anatomic variance during occiput—C2 fusion. (A) Preoperative CTA in patient undergoing occiput—C2 fusion with axial view of C2 showing narrow left pedicle and anomalous medialized left VA. (B) Intraoperative lateral view of the final occiput—C2 fusion construct. (C) Right-sided fixation performed with translaminar screw to avoid narrow pedicle and anomalous VA. (D) C2 pedicle screw placed in larger right-sided pedicle.

importance. Initial response should include direct tamponade or pressure over the bleeding surface to reduce bleeding. In the posterior subaxial spine this may occur simply with placement of a screw into the screw hole or bone wax. The authors would advocate for placement of a short screw into the screw hole to allow for the benefits of fixation as well as tamponade. If the vessel is injured during the approach in the atlantoaxial spine or in the anterior cervical spine with direct laceration, the use of hemostatic agents including oxycellulose for example, Surgicel (Ethicon) or absorbable gelatin sponges for example, Gelfoam (Pfizer) may be helpful to gain initial hemostasis. Large bore suctions should be used at this time to allow for visualization and evacuation of blood from the field to allow for identification of the source and tamponade.

Ideally, a microvascular set is available in all cases, particularly those in the anterior cervical spine where direct access to the VA is possible. This set should include vessel clips, aneurysm clips, micro forceps, microsuction tips, and needle drivers to allow for the handling of small sutures such as 6 to 0 through 8 to 0 polypropylene suture.

Team Considerations
At the onset, the anesthesia team should be alerted to the potential of a major vascular injury to allow for appropriate resuscitative measures including the maintenance of appropriate blood pressure parameters with the use of vasopressors and blood product administration. Case studies have listed maintaining mean arterial pressures of 90 to 100 mm Hg to optimize collateral perfusion to the vertebrobasilar area in the setting of VAIs.[18]

In addition, arrangements should be made to obtain intraoperative consultation with vascular surgery, neurovascular surgery, or neurointerventional radiology as this injury is fairly rare and will require additional expertise. Enlistment of an additional spine surgeon, particularly a senior colleague, may be helpful for experience and assistance in complication management.

Exposure
In the anterior cervical spine, exposure and repair is an option for iatrogenic VAI. Exposure of the ipsilateral VA is generally straightforward through the initial approach incision; however, the contralateral VA may be difficult to access and may require a mirror incision. Access to the VA can either be performed by dissection of the sternocleidomastoid laterally or, more commonly, extending the anterior cervical

approach in a lateral direction, revealing the lateral border of the uncinate processes and the VA traveling through the lateral foramen. It is possible to palpate the costal process that houses the VA. Longus colli should be dissected from the costal process from medial to lateral to avoid sympathetic chain injury. The intertransverse membrane can be dissected with a curette or bipolar cautery. The anterior branch of the transverse process should then be removed using a 2 mm Kerrison rongeur or burr depending on familiarity and comfort. In addition, it is generally easier to move from superior to inferior based on the angle of the process. Depending on the type of injury to the VA, complete transection may result in the retraction of one side or both sides of the artery requiring further cranial or caudal dissection.

Once visualization of the VA is achieved, bipolar cautery is used for the surrounding venous plexus and distal and proximal control is obtained using temporary clips or vessel loops. Care must be taken as the cervical nerve roots run just deep to the artery as it is possible to also produce a nerve root injury. The authors would emphasize that exposure of the VA should be attempted several times in a cadaver lab to allow for familiarity in dealing with this complication. Although there may be some consideration of primary repair from a posterior subaxial approach, significant dissection and bony work would limit its utility.[19]

Once control of the bleeding has been obtained, it can be followed by definitive treatment either with ligation or repair.

Consideration of Direct Repair or Ligation
In the event neurointerventional radiology/surgery and vascular surgery are not immediately available, several factors will guide treatment. The first consideration will be the artery dominance. This should be generally determined from preoperative imaging. After gaining control of both the cranial and caudal aspect of the VA, it is possible to evaluate the potential artery dominance. If the superior vessel is released and bleeding is present, this suggests a patent circle of Willis or intact collateral circulation and it is possible to ligate the artery without significant consequence. However, if with release of the superior vessel, no bleeding is present; this suggests that the injured artery is dominant and it is preferable to directly repair the vessel to prevent ischemic complications.[14] Choice of management is heavily affected by the circumstances of surgery, availability of other specialists, and clinical status of the patient.

Direct Repair

Microsurgical repair is then carried out using 6 to 0 through 8 to 0 polypropylene sutures using microinstruments as the artery is typically around 6 cm deep to the skin. Small side tears can be repaired using simple interrupted or figure-of-eight sutures. Larger tears may require interposition graft or patch. Patency after repair should be confirmed with angiography or Doppler.[20] In a systematic review, Guan and colleagues[14] found that no secondary management was required and no complications were observed in patients undergoing direct repair of the VA.

Ligation and Angiography

At times, direct repair may not be a feasible option and occlusion of the artery to definitively control hemorrhage may be necessary. Both suture ligation and vascular clips are options for open occlusion of the vessel. However, if possible, urgent intraoperative angiography should be performed to assess vessel dominance and collateral flow.[14,21] If there is adequate collateral flow, occlusion via vascular clips or suture ligation is a valid option. This assessment is imperative to outcomes as ligation without knowing vascular dominance can lead to a reported complication rate of 43% and mortality rate of 12%. When performing ligation it is still important to obtain proper visualization of the injured vessel to avoid injuring the cervical nerve roots. Patients undergoing ligation were at risk for nerve root injury, whereas patients undergoing embolization were at risk for infarction in a literature review by Guan and colleagues.[14] Endovascular occlusion via embolization or occlusion is another option when available which bypasses this risk. However, if there is inadequate collateral flow on angiography, open reconstruction or endovascular stenting, or possible flow diversion in the setting of a pseudoaneurysm should be attempted to avoid ischemic injury. The patient should be admitted to an intensive care unit postoperatively for close monitoring and further evaluation for additional vascular pathology with advanced imaging.[21]

Avoidance of Further Complications

Emboli leading to cerebral infarction can result from injury or intervention on an injured VA. When ligating or using vascular clips, it is essential to intervene on both the proximal and distal aspects of the vessel. This will help avoid delayed embolic or hemorrhagic complications as well as formation of arterio-venous fistulas. These complications can arise from addressing only the proximal limb of the vessel.[22]

Unilateral VA should prompt extreme caution with instrumentation of the contralateral side, particularly if only the nondominant side is injured.[23] Deep subfascial drain placement is recommended, particularly in the anterior cervical spine to avoid any potential complication relating to retropharyngeal hematoma.

Postoperative Management

Postoperative evaluation with angiography, CT angiogram, or MR angiogram should be performed. In addition, vascular or neurointerventional radiology/surgery consultation should be attained, especially in circumstances where the surgeon is unable to directly repair or ligate the vessel.[15] Guan and colleagues[14] found in 25 patients in which hemorrhage control was obtained via tamponade and packing. Twelve patients (48%) developed a pseudoaneurysm and 5 of these patients experienced hemorrhage in the acute postop period. These patients required secondary management with either coiling, stenting, or repair. Complications in patients who underwent this method of management included pharyngeal discomfort, swallowing difficulty, lateral medullary syndrome, and cerebral infarction.

In addition, AVF is also possible.[24] However, a normal angiogram immediately postoperatively does not rule out the risk of further complications. Complications can occur days to months after the initial insult.[14] Despite this limitation, Mwipatayi and colleagues[25] found postoperative angiography to be an effective diagnostic tool while also allowing for timely intervention in a review of 151 patients with VAIs.[15] Depending on the type of vascular injury, collateral circulation, and morphology of the Circle of Willis, consideration would be made for either stent placement or coil to allow for either maintained flow or to sacrifice the vessel, respectively. In addition, the authors recommend postoperative mean arterial pressure above 90 mm Hg in the interim time period following suspected injury to ensure adequate cerebral perfusion.[18]

Medical Therapies

First-line medical management for patients who are asymptomatic from a VAI consists of close observation and antiplatelet or anticoagulation therapy. Neither antiplatelet nor anticoagulation therapy has been established to be superior in prevention of complications from VAI. Anticoagulation therapy typically consists of heparin, whereas antiplatelet therapy is typically aspirin. The CADISS study (Cervical Artery in Dissection Stroke Study) was a randomized controlled trial comparing antiplatelet versus anticoagulation therapy in the treatment of extracranial VA dissection. The study consisted of 126 patients treated with antiplatelet therapy and 124 patients treated with anticoagulation therapy. Three patients in the antiplatelet group suffered death or stroke, whereas 1 patient in the anticoagulation group suffered a stroke. No statistically significant difference was detected among the 2 modalities.[26,27] A deep subfascial drain should be placed intraoperatively in patients with suspected VAI. Although the vascular complication is the most life-threatening, a retropharyngeal hematoma while initiating any form of anticoagulation may compound the issue with the possibility of airway compromise.

Complications

Fortunately, the risk of neurologic sequelae from unilateral VAI and ischemia is relatively low at 2.7% to 6.7%. This is due to collateral perfusion by the other VA and the communicating posterior communicating arteries.[19] However, catastrophic consequences can occur as a direct result of the insult including thrombosis, transient ischemic attack, stroke, and death. Angiography showing normal status of an injured VA does not rule out subsequent formation of pseudoaneurysm and delayed hemorrhage. Cases of pseudoaneurysm and bleeding have been reported days to years later.[28,29] Delayed hemorrhage or embolic infarcts due to these vascular abnormalities are possible.

Patients suspected to have sustained iatrogenic VAI should be followed by angiography to evaluate vessel anatomy and exclude growing pseudoaneurysm. Evaluation should be performed in the late periods as well. The authors would recommend postoperative cerebral angiogram as soon as possible, followed by CT angiogram at 1 week. Based on the injury and method of intervention, this can be followed with successive imaging at various time points (in discussion with vascular subspecialists). Considerations for follow-up imaging include evaluating for possible propagation of a dissection or growth of a pseudoaneurysm in the case these are not treated. Fistulous communication between the VA and its surrounding plexus following VAI has been described in several case series. There are few reports describing this complication from anterior cervical surgery.[28,30] Different management strategies have been proposed with most authors favoring primary repair of the vessel whenever possible. Neurologic sequelae may occur following direct ligation or coils of the collateral vessels if flow is unable to be maintained by a hypoplastic contralateral artery.

Pseudoaneurysms or AVFs can be treated with endovascular techniques including coil embolization, stent-assisted coil embolization, self-expandable stenting, covered stents, or flow diverter placement.[24,29,31] Spinal AVF can be similarly treated by transarterial or venous approaches.

SUMMARY

Iatrogenic VAI is a rare but potentially catastrophic complication. Advanced imaging techniques and increased anatomic knowledge are crucial to the prevention of these complications during cervical spine surgeries performed for various cervical spine disorders. Regardless of the surgical approach, surgeons must be aware of the potential for VAI and take the necessary steps for prevention of complications by understanding a patient's vascular anatomy, recognizing anatomic anomalies, undertaking proper surgical planning, and maintaining close monitoring during the perioperative period. Surgeons must be aware of the appropriate management strategies for VAI and be prepared to perform hemostatic tamponade, microvascular repair, or anastomosis as needed. VA dominance and collateral circulation must be known preoperatively before surgical ligation or permanent clipping is attempted. Recent advancements in endovascular treatment have provided increased intervention options in iatrogenic VAI. In the event of VAI, local control of bleeding is the first concern followed by immediate angiography, serial endovascular treatment, and close monitoring of the patient.

CLINICS CARE POINTS

- Iatrogenic vertebral artery injury (VAI) is a rare but potentially devastating complication of cervical spine surgery.

- Surgeons should be aware of anatomic variants of the vertebral artery, the presence of which can be detected on meticulous review of preoperative imaging.

- Prevention is key to avoiding any injury through knowledge of patient anatomy, procedure and instrumentation selection, care in dissection, and meticulous surgical technique.

- Initial management of VAI includes tamponade and enlistment of anesthesia assistance in addition to neurointerventional radiology/surgery or vascular surgery if available.

- Treatment modalities remain controversial and include tamponade, direct repair, ligation, or endovascular interventions.
- Surgeons must be aware of late complications of VAI such as delayed hemorrhage, pseudoaneurysm, and arteriovenous fistula in addition to management options.

DISCLOSURE

The authors have nothing to disclose.

ACKNOWLEDGMENTS

The authors sincerely thank the artist, Jacqueline Cabessa Redlich, for providing the original artwork used in the article.

REFERENCES

1. Yi HJ. Epidemiology and Management of Iatrogenic Vertebral Artery Injury Associated With Cervical Spine Surgery. Korean J Nutr 2022;18(1):34–44.
2. Inamasu J, Guiot BH. Iatrogenic vertebral artery injury. Acta Neurol Scand 2005;112(6):349–57.
3. Curylo LJ, Mason HC, Bohlman HH, et al. Tortuous course of the vertebral artery and anterior cervical decompression: a cadaveric and clinical case study. Spine 2000;25(22):2860–4.
4. Hong JM, Chung CS, Bang OY, et al. Vertebral artery dominance contributes to basilar artery curvature and peri-vertebrobasilar junctional infarcts. J Neurol Neurosurg Psychiatry 2009;80(10):1087–92.
5. Bruneau M, Cornelius JF, Marneffe V, et al. Anatomical Variations of the V2 Segment of the Vertebral Artery. Neurosurgery 2006;59(1). https://doi.org/10.1227/01.NEU.0000219931.64378.B5.ONS-20.
6. Eskander MS, Drew JM, Aubin ME, et al. Vertebral Artery Anatomy: A Review of Two Hundred Fifty Magnetic Resonance Imaging Scans. Spine 2010;35(23):2035–40.
7. Park JH, Kim JM, Roh JK. Hypoplastic vertebral artery: frequency and associations with ischaemic stroke territory. J Neurol Neurosurg Psychiatry 2007;78(9):954–8.
8. Ergun O, Gunes Tatar I, Birgi E, et al. Evaluation of vertebral artery dominance, hypoplasia and variations in the origin: angiographic study in 254 patients. Folia Morphol (Warsz) 2016;75(1):33–7.
9. Uchino A, Saito N, Watadani T, et al. Vertebral artery variations at the C1-2 level diagnosed by magnetic resonance angiography. Neuroradiology 2012;54(1):19–23.
10. Sarmiento JM, Cohen JD, Babadjouni RM, et al. Evaluation of tortuous vertebral arteries before cervical spine surgery: illustrative case. J Neurosurg Case Lessons 2021;1(20). CASE2198.
11. Zhang H. Preoperative Imaging Evaluation to Safeguard Anomalous Vertebral Artery in Posterior C2 Fixation. OSMOAJ 2020;3(4). https://doi.org/10.32474/OSMOAJ.2020.03.000166.
12. Elliott RE, Tanweer O, Boah A, et al. Comparison of screw malposition and vertebral artery injury of C2 pedicle and transarticular screws: meta-analysis and review of the literature. J Spinal Disord Tech 2014;27(6):305–15.
13. Oga M, Yuge I, Terada K, et al. Tortuosity of the vertebral artery in patients with cervical spondylotic myelopathy. Risk factor for the vertebral artery injury during anterior cervical decompression. Spine 1996;21(9):1085–9.
14. Guan Q, Chen L, Long Y, et al. Iatrogenic Vertebral Artery Injury During Anterior Cervical Spine Surgery: A Systematic Review. World Neurosurg 2017;106:715–22.
15. Ghaith AK, Yolcu YU, Alvi MA, et al. Rate and Characteristics of Vertebral Artery Injury Following C1-C2 Posterior Cervical Fusion: A Systematic Review and Meta-Analysis. World Neurosurg 2021;148:118–26.
16. Young JP, Young PH, Ackermann MJ, et al. The ponticulus posticus: implications for screw insertion into the first cervical lateral mass. J Bone Joint Surg Am 2005;87(11):2495–8.
17. Coe JD, Vaccaro AR, Dailey AT, et al. Lateral mass screw fixation in the cervical spine: a systematic literature review. J Bone Joint Surg Am 2013;95(23):2136–43.
18. Paramaswamy R. Airway management in a displaced comminuted fracture of the mandible and atlas with a vertebral artery injury: A case report. J Dent Anesth Pain Med 2018;18(3):183–7.
19. Wright NM, Lauryssen C. Vertebral artery injury in C1-2 transarticular screw fixation: results of a survey of the AANS/CNS section on disorders of the spine and peripheral nerves. American Association of Neurological Surgeons/Congress of Neurological Surgeons. J Neurosurg 1998;88(4):634–40.
20. Belykh E, Xu DS, Yağmurlu K, et al. Repair of V2 Vertebral Artery Injuries Sustained During Anterior Cervical Diskectomy. World Neurosurg 2017;105:796–804.
21. Ramamurti P, Weinreb J, Fassihi SC, et al. Vertebral Artery Injury in the Cervical Spine: Anatomy, Diagnosis, and Management. JBJS Rev 2021;9(1). e20.00118.
22. Golfinos JG, Dickman CA, Zabramski JM, et al. Repair of vertebral artery injury during anterior cervical decompression. Spine 1994;19(22):2552–6.
23. Finn MA, Apfelbaum RI. Atlantoaxial transarticular screw fixation: update on technique and outcomes

in 269 patients. Neurosurgery 2010;66(3 Suppl): 184–92.

24. Lo WB, Nagaraja S, Saxena A. Delayed Hemorrhage from an Iatrogenic Vertebral Artery Injury During Anterior Cervical Discectomy and Successful Endovascular Treatment-Report of a Rare Case and Literature Review. World Neurosurg 2017;99: 811. e11-811.e18.

25. Mwipatayi BP, Jeffery P, Beningfield SJ, et al. Management of extra-cranial vertebral artery injuries. Eur J Vasc Endovasc Surg 2004;27(2):157–62.

26. Hall M, Cheng D, Cheng W, et al. Antiplatelet versus Anticoagulation for Asymptomatic Patients with Vertebral Artery Injury during Anterior Cervical Surgery-Two Case Reports and Review of Literature. Brain Sci 2019;9(12):345.

27. Caplan LR. Antiplatelets vs anticoagulation for dissection: CADISS nonrandomized arm and meta-analysis. Neurology 2013;80(10):970–1.

28. Cosgrove GR, Théron J. Vertebral arteriovenous fistula following anterior cervical spine surgery. Report of two cases. J Neurosurg 1987;66(2):297–9.

29. Choi JW, Lee JK, Moon KS, et al. Endovascular embolization of iatrogenic vertebral artery injury during anterior cervical spine surgery: report of two cases and review of the literature. Spine 2006;31(23):E891–4.

30. Daentzer D, Deinsberger W, Böker DK. Vertebral artery complications in anterior approaches to the cervical spine: report of two cases and review of literature. Surg Neurol 2003;59(4):300–9 [discussion: 309].

31. Garcia Alzamora M, Rosahl SK, Lehmberg J, et al. Life-threatening bleeding from a vertebral artery pseudoaneurysm after anterior cervical spine approach: endovascular repair by a triple stent-in-stent method. Case report. Neuroradiology 2005; 47(4):282–6.

Moving?

Make sure your subscription moves with you!

To notify us of your new address, find your **Clinics Account Number** (located on your mailing label above your name), and contact customer service at:

Email: journalscustomerservice-usa@elsevier.com

800-654-2452 (subscribers in the U.S. & Canada)
314-447-8871 (subscribers outside of the U.S. & Canada)

Fax number: 314-447-8029

Elsevier Health Sciences Division
Subscription Customer Service
3251 Riverport Lane
Maryland Heights, MO 63043

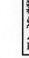

Printed and bound by CPI Group (UK) Ltd, Croydon, CR0 4YY

08/05/2025

01864750-0019